Praise for Peter Nielsen and *Will of Iron*

"I've always believed that anything in life is possible and Peter Nielsen is a great testimonial to that belief."
—Jack LaLanne, the "Godfather of Physical Fitness"

"I've trained with Peter for a number of years and reaped great benefits from his knowledge and attitude. The main ideas he lays out in this book—nutrition, exercise, and mental attitude—are the perfect recipe for success, in my sport or any athletic training. The first thing I learned from Peter was to think critically about the food I put into my body and how it affects my training. To get the performance I expect of myself out there on the ice, I have to keep my body tuned like a machine—and nutrition is definitely the master fuel. I use the same nutrition principles outlined in this book to get that advantage. But probably the most extraordinary aspect about Peter's principles is his message about positive mental attitude. He is at the top of my list when it comes to positive motivation and inspiration. If you are looking for serious motivation and a solid fitness message, read this book—you will walk away fired up to be the best you can."
—Darren McCarty, Detroit Red Wing and three-time NHL Stanley Cup Champion

"I have known Peter for a good many years and I can confirm that his principles on health and fitness apply to people of all ages. Peter and I have worked together on a number of occasions, during which time I have gained a great deal of confidence in his message and ability to effectively communicate these powerful concepts to others. Peter's teaching on proper nutrition and regular exercise is invaluable, and something that I, too, have tried to emphasize throughout my career. I have always said that a healthy diet and a fit body are key elements for success. My advice to everyone is to get this book, apply these principles and start living life to its fullest!"
—Gary Player, Professional Golfer and Winner of Golf's Grand Slam

"Peter Nielsen's principles of nutrition and fitness have helped me consistently over the years. The routines he outlines in this book are part of a jump-start program he put me on a few years ago. I went from off-season shape to peak muscle definition and energy levels in six weeks. I continue to turn back to that same program whenever I want to achieve maximum physical condition."
—Joe Montana, Pro Football Hall of Famer

Will of Iron
Principles for Healthy Living

Peter N. Nielsen
with Tom Ferguson and Roseanna Zia

Momentum Books LLC
Royal Oak, Michigan

Cover photo by Chris Scalise

Manufactured in the United States of America

2005   2004   2003   5   4   3   2   1

Momentum Books LLC
117 W. Third Street
Royal Oak, Michigan 48067

ISBN 1-879094-69-X

Library of Congress Control Number: 2003105274

Nielsen, Peter, 1961—

       Will of iron : principles for healthy living /
Peter Nielsen.
       p.   cm.

ISBN 1-879094-69-X (pbk.) : $19.95

1. Exercise. 2. Physical fitness. 3. Health. I. Title.

To Pete and Marie,
who gave me my good name;

To Cindy,
who accepted it
and who has unconditionally loved me,
through good times and bad;

And to my children,
who have taught a grown man how to truly love;
through whose eyes I have learned
the words humility and humbleness;
and who have given me the gift to be childlike again.

Table of Contents

AUTHOR'S PREFACE   IX
INTRODUCTION   I

PART ONE: SCARS AND BARBELLS

1 A WORLD TURNED INSIDE OUT   13
2 THE BRIDGE   21
3 "THEY LOOK LIKE TOOTHPICKS"   29
4 TROPHY TIME   37
5 MUSCLE GLITZ   45
6 NEW LIFE IN MOTOWN   51
7 ATTITUDE—THE KEY THAT TURNS EVERY LOCK   61

PART TWO: NUTRITION: WHERE IT ALL BEGINS

8   GOING AGAINST THE FLOW   67
9   WHAT'S IN IT FOR ME?   77
10 NOT WEIGHT LOSS, BUT FAT LOSS   97
11 FUELING FOR PERFORMANCE   107
12 THE BUILDING BLOCK FOR MUSCLE   117
13 SO WHAT'S ON THE MENU?   121
14 NUTRITION AND KIDS (ADULTS, LISTEN UP)   131

PART THREE: SWEAT EQUITY

15 Starting at Square One 137
16 Conditioning, Plain and Simple 143
17 You Gotta Have Heart 149
18 Anatomy of a Workout 157
19 Five Levels, Five Programs 167
20 Going All the Way 181
21 Fighting a Flabby Future 187

PART FOUR: MENTAL DISCIPLINE

22 Commitment and that Inner Fire 197
23 The Game Plan 205
24 Me vs. Me 209
25 You Gotta Have a Plan 213
26 Getting Ready for Battle 217
27 Charting Your Course 229
28 Seize the Miracle 237

Acknowledgements 241

Resources 245

Author's Preface

In life there is always opportunity. Sometimes we see it; sometimes we are too afraid to see it. Opportunity often comes in the form of adversity or challenge—and therein lies the rub.

At the time I didn't realize it, but as I look back now, I've been blessed with the opportunity to be a vehicle to touch the lives of many people. These are people of every sort—from persons with physical handicaps or serious health challenges to elite athletes at the apex of their sports.

It has always been my desire to help people learn from the experiences and mistakes of others—including myself. One lesson I learned painfully was that, as Albert Einstein said, inside every catastrophe lies opportunity. The quality of my life is due in great part to blessings that came from situations that seemed disastrous when they were happening. I discovered that when you are in a situation that can't be avoided but must be dealt with, it is the *attitude* you take that separates the survivors from the victims, the champions from the defeated.

Those challenges, the bad moments in life, are opportunities to make something more and better of ourselves. For me, responding to adversity took the form of building a healthier lifestyle. Much of what I have discovered on my journey was learned from others.

I want to light in others the same spark that has been kindled in me—the spark that saved my life.

But as much as I wanted to share these insights and concepts with others, I realized that I couldn't do it alone. In the first release of this book, it was my great good fortune to meet up with Tom Ferguson, a person with the skill and determination to wade through the first 31 years of my life and shape it into the story on these pages. His talent is considerable and is exceeded only by his qualities as a person.

Ten years of good living passed since that first release, and have added a dimension to my perspective that demanded an update and re-release of this book. Good fortune again crossed my path in the form of Roseanna Zia. Along with updates to my story, we've added a new Introduction and several new chapters that present the best and newest of my message of health, fitness and lifestyle. Roseanna's passion and zest for life are contagious. The crossroads in her own life have made her who she is today. Her energy has opened up my mind and spirit. And in return, she enabled me to express my heart and soul on paper. It was a blessing that our paths have crossed.

If this book speaks to you or touches you in any way—and I fervently hope that it does—then we both owe thanks to my collaborators, Tom Ferguson and Roseanna Zia.

P.N.N.
May 2003

Introduction

I don't look like a person who spends his life behind a desk or on the couch, who smokes, eats fast food five times a week, and hasn't lifted anything heavier than the remote control in 15 years. More importantly, I don't *feel* like one.

I look and feel like someone who gets 24 good hours out of each and every day, and who is thrilled to be alive. I can't wait to get started on my day. I don't run out of energy, I run out of *clock*.

The interesting and sad part is that the average person probably considers *me* to be the oddball. Because I pay serious attention to the one and only fragile frame that will carry me from cradle to grave. Because I'm more aware of what I eat than what's on television tonight. Because I take better care of myself than I do my car—and believe me, my car is in mint condition. And because I'm a bodybuilder.

Does the first person I described above sound a little too much like you? Does it give you a tug of guilt or sadness because you are more like the first person, but wish you were more like the second? Does it make you feel like you are letting yourself down?

If so, read on. Because you *are* letting yourself down. And you can change that.

This book isn't about trying to convince you that every American should be down at the gym this afternoon pumping iron and bench-pressing the equivalent of their body weight, or that your entire life should revolve around the gym and rice cakes, or some super-special diet and fitness routine.

I am writing this book because when I look around me, I see a society filled with people dragging through life in impaired, exhausted bodies. Occasionally I see a spark where a person glimpses their true healthy, energetic potential. But the spark is soon snuffed out by exhausting schedules,

1

the incredible cheapness of incredibly unhealthy food, and a world full of drive-ins, drive-ups, drive-thrus and cable TV with remote. People race to the weekend hoping to get in a little "quality time," but there is so little quality in their physical condition, they barely have the energy to enjoy it. And yet they don't seize the opportunity to change it.

The only question you I have for you is: Are *you* ready for change?

It distresses me that human nature seems to require crisis before action—a fatal crash before a streetlight is installed or a massive coronary before the cigarettes and junk food get tossed aside. And I am absolutely, passionately convinced that *it doesn't have to take a crisis for you to wake up and change your life for the better.*

Believe me, your body does not care what color you are, how much money you have, how beautiful you are, what car you drive, or what your address is. If it wants your attention, one way or another, it's going to get it. And if you ignore it, well, the wakeup calls just get louder and louder.

I got my wakeup call as a teenager, when a disabling illness nearly took my life. Physical fitness was my way up and out. At the time, all I was doing was trying to save my life, and I had a shred of hope that I might do it with a healthy body. Very little was known about treating my disease. All I knew was that every piece of food I put in my mouth was either nutrition or poison, and that exercise was medicine. I didn't get healthy because it was the "right" thing to do. I got healthy because it was the *only* thing to do. And it worked, far beyond just keeping me alive.

In the years that followed my seemingly miraculous recovery, I took step after step along a path that brought me ever-higher levels of health. And it wasn't long before fitness healed more than my body—it healed my whole life. Being physically healthy taught me to care for my body. Caring *for* my body taught me to care *about* my body. And caring about my body taught me the most surprising part of all—how to care about *me.*

And that led to my tremendous passion for helping others in the same way.

Are you caring for *your* body? Do you care *about* your body? About yourself? Are these questions foreign to you? If you walked over to the mirror right now and looked at it, would you cringe? Would you be looking at a body that you only tolerate, even reject? If you do, you need to keep reading. But first, I want to introduce you to someone.

Go back to that mirror, take a good long look, and say hello. You are looking at your best friend and most loyal defender. It's the only body you'll be issued. Are you ready to make friends with your lifelong partner? If you are, read on. If you're not sure, *read on.*

I'm not talking about winning a weightlifting trophy—I'm talking about feeling, looking and living better than you ever have before.

My main concern in writing this book has nothing to do with athleticism, or with muscular bodies than can be oiled up and displayed on a stage. It has everything to do with all the more important things that are *affected* by our physical condition. Those things include family life, self-esteem, longevity, career, sexual health and earning power. I am going to focus on connecting the dots—the cause and effect—between a healthy body and a healthy life. It's all about how taking care of your health makes you take better care of every part of your life.

I am often called a "fitness guru." I'll own that. Years of experimentation with my own body and a display case full of championship trophies (all achieved drug-free) tell me that, yeah, I know what I'm doing when it comes to fitness and nutrition. But I also get a little uneasy about the word "guru." It implies that I know something that is beyond most people and they have to come up to the mountaintop to find it out. My message is just the opposite.

My goal is to light your inner fire—and teach *you* how to keep it burning. Of all the thousands of things that no one else can do for you, physical fitness is at the very top of the list. You can buy a personal trainer, but he cannot do your exercises. Even if you could afford to keep him around seven days a week, he cannot force you to make the right eating choices. Even if he could be with you 24 hours a day, leading you through every step of nutrition and exercise, you would miss out on the amazing self-confidence and self-respect that come from caring directly for yourself. And those things are half the benefit! Fitness is about quality of life—not just muscles.

So, let's address a few of the inevitable "bodybuilder" misconceptions that often come up. The reason I want to speak to this is that as human beings, we constantly get a mental picture of who we are, what our identity is. Plain and simple, you don't have to be Mr. or Ms. Universe to build your body. Let's sweep away stereotypes right off the bat. They usually go something like this:

"He must be a real egomaniac to want to look like that."

"He has more biceps than brains."

"He got a little help at the drugstore."

Are there bodybuilders or fitness enthusiasts out there who fit these descriptions? Sure. Just like plumbers, lawyers, students and world leaders, there are great examples and there are poor examples. I can only speak for myself.

Being deeply grateful for the life I have and being an egomaniac are two states of mind that are not compatible. I spend far more time on the gratitude end of the scale than most people I know. As I hinted earlier, as an adolescent I faced challenges that, physically, emotionally and mentally, I could hardly meet. I had two choices: Give in, give up and get bitter, or get up, get strong and get better. I believe that the choices we make far out-weigh the circumstances that are thrown at us in life. That belief is respon-sible for a lot of my success. And I earned that belief—it didn't come easily. I had a Hand on my shoulder as I carved my path, and somewhere inside I promised I would try to give it back. Ego has very little to do with it for me.

Barbells for brains? My wife says I'm smarter than the average bear, but she may be a little biased. Somehow, though, I'm managing a thriving personal training club, a state-of-the-art fitness center, a busy appearance schedule, syndicated television and radio shows, and a very active Web site. For some reason in our culture, we assume you can be a strong athlete or a solid intel-lect, but not both. I value being both, and so can you. I'm not going to tell you that being fit will make you a genius. Yet I know that a mind supported by exercise and good nutrition is sharper than an exhausted, starved one.

Drugs and bodybuilding is a very serious issue, and I have a totally black-and-white position on the subject. Supporting bodybuilding with drugs is dangerous and unacceptable. I got into the sport of bodybuilding to save my life, not flush it down a drain; I turned to bodybuilding to nurture a struggling body, not to poison it. Also, bodybuilding is about finding the best within yourself, not about tricking your body into it with drugs. My gym is filled with trophies I won "clean" before retiring in 1984. The main reason I came out of retirement in 1991 was that my sport finally commis-sioned a sanctioning body that administers blood, urine and polygraph tests to all competitors. I have always competed clean and drug-free, and now that fact can be officially certified.

Besides these stereotypes, there is another common misperception: the idea that in bodybuilding, there is no middle ground. The truth is, you don't have to go for the Mr. Universe title or be able to do one-handed pushups to make a big change in your health. Let me explain.

Pros are supposed to be exaggerated examples of skill and talent. For example, I have always loved to watch Gary Player golf. And even though my game is nowhere near the same solar system as his, I still enjoy golf. He taps that little white golf ball around the course like it takes personal instruction from him. He happens to be gifted, and he has dedicated the better part of his life honing his skill. The fact that most of us could never achieve his level of play does not stop us from golfing and getting immense pleasure out of more modest accomplishments. After all, what would the world be like if none of us played football because we couldn't be Joe Montana, or none of us played tennis because we couldn't all be Venus or Serena Williams?

So you can still use me as an example. Sure, I'm big, and my musculature is unusually well defined. I'm a pro—I'm *supposed* to look like that. I've spent the better part of my life fine-tuning my body. Could I have an immensely fulfilling life with half the dedication and none of the titles? Definitely. But I spend time in the gym every day building muscle because I enjoy it, and I make my living at it; I treat food like a prescription drug because for me, it is. You can get phenomenal results without going *one-tenth* as far as I did, just by using the same principles.

Now that we know that you don't have to be Mr. Monster Biceps or Wonder Woman to focus on your health, what *are* the types of people out there building their bodies?

My fitness centers are filled with bodybuilders of both sexes, all ages and endless shapes and sizes. The range of clientele would stagger your mind. We have major-league hockey and basketball players, automotive company executives, professionals, teachers, hairstylists, salespeople, stay-at-home parents, teenagers, retirees, and more. Some pay the fee out of their pocket money; some have to budget tightly for this commitment to their health.

And yes, some of our bodybuilders have physiques that require them to buy their clothing custom-made. The majority of them, however, don't stand out in a crowd—which is exactly their goal.

Tara Terrell, for instance, is a bodybuilder. She has lupus. Tara works out almost every day. She doesn't want to build a stage physique. She just wants to get her health back, to be "normal."

Chuck Robertson is a successful businessman, the owner of a swimming pool company. He has a very rare, debilitating disease that is attacking all of his muscles—even his tongue. He works out constantly to fight the atrophy and to keep the disease in remission. Chuck is a bodybuilder, one of the gutsiest I've ever met.

So if you take a look at the bodybuilding scene, the reality is that there are two stereotypes—one group of bodies that you more or less had pictured, and one group of bodies that you probably hadn't.

Unfortunately, most bodybuilders fit one stereotype or the other—advanced practitioners of the sport, or fragile human beings who have found that their last, best chance lies in a serious physical regimen.

Either way, they are *building their bodies*. Getting healthier. Raising confidence and self-esteem. Nothing odd about that.

So let's clear that misconception away before we even get out of the gate. Remember that mirror we talked about? You don't have to look into it and try to see a Greek god or goddess; a fitness lifestyle does not mean a sudden transformation to a muscle-bound gym rat. It means that you get to define your own goals, then pick the point where you'd like to be—and together, we'll get there.

You will hear me get passionate about my message—I may even get a little preachy. I'll own that, because I *am* passionate about my message—health, fitness and lifestyle! If you want to be a serious bodybuilder, that's great. You'll learn a lot in the pages of this book, including some bona fide secrets of a champion. But you can get a lot out of this book *even if you never set foot in a gym.*

That's a lead-in to the third major misconception: Most people believe that to get a firm, healthy, fit body with solid, flexible muscles, you need fancy gym equipment or a gym membership. You don't. As a veteran gym-member and current club owner myself, I can tell you that gyms don't have a patent on exercise, or even on bodybuilding. I worked out at home for a year and a half before even setting foot in a gym. Give me a set of free-weights, a mat and a pair of sneakers, and I'll hand you a thorough and challenging workout.

And contrary to what you might think, competitive bodybuilding is just as much a matter of nutrition and mental focus as it is a matter of pumping iron. I'm in my early forties, and I work out about an hour a day. I haven't lost any muscle mass since my last Mr. Universe title. Yet every step I make in muscle development now comes *more* from the kitchen than from the gym; *more* from the brain than from the sweat glands. What that means for you is that more than 60 percent of the improvement in your health and physique will come from what you put in your mouth. Any unintelligent person can pump iron—lifting a barbell is not rocket science. But effective nutrition truly is science—plus, it takes real self-discipline at the breakfast, lunch and dinner table to pull off a fit and healthy lifestyle.

There is a lot to be said for the focus of working out alone at home, but just as much can be said for the synergy you get from working out around other people with the same goal. I've learned a lot from the many exercisers, trainers and clients that I have met in gyms through the years. Gyms and health clubs can also be a great way to experiment with lots of aerobic equipment and classes as well, especially in those really hot or really frigid months. You can get the full range of fitness exercises.

I like to convey to people that fitness is more than lifting weights. It's that, plus flexibility, cardiovascular fitness, nutrition and even stress man-agement. Both of my fitness clubs are called "Total Fitness Centers" for just that reason. Some of our clients just want to come in and lift weights. That's OK. But I also offer nutrition counseling, advice on training pro-grams and, sometimes, just a good talk about the commitment to self that it takes to bring out your best. We have an aerobics circuit and I try to get even our best lifters involved with it. Why? Because if you can bench-press the Empire State Building but you're sucking wind walking up two flights of stairs, you are not in good shape!

So this business of fitness is a *total* package, just like life. My life's total package is made up of my wife and children, my family, my faith, my health, my friends, my fitness message, my career, and my athletic ability—I don't know if you could find a more grateful man than me.

Keeping the life package together depends on maintaining all of those key areas, especially your health. If you take care of each piece of the total package, it helps support the rest. For example, attending church does not bring home my paycheck, but the lessons I learn and the peace I find there definitely sustain me in my daily pursuits. Loving my wife and children does not make people tune in to my radio or television programs—but part of why my audience likes who they see and hear comes from the caring, grounded, satisfied person my family makes me. Being physically fit does not run my businesses or manage my employees. But my fitness lifestyle stokes and strengthens my body, keeping me on my toes through all of the day's business, leaving me energized at the end of a jam-packed week. Every piece is interconnected.

I can guarantee you that if you walk away from any key piece of the total package, every other part will suffer. If you get obsessed with working out or pumping iron, your life will get lopsided. If you have no fitness focus at all, your life will get lopsided. Either way, you're not evenly yoked, and any team of horses not evenly yoked struggles and eventually stumbles.

You can't afford to ignore fitness. Unfortunately, most people feel so overwhelmed in their lives that they don't think they have *time* for fitness.

That's why most Americans fall somewhere into the vast, flabby middle ground between Mr./Ms. Universe and Mr./Ms. Couch-Potato-Remote-Controller. Fitness is something they want to be involved in, but can't seem to make time for. They make well intentioned but humorous stabs at it—ordering diet soda with their french fries, or eating frozen yogurt instead of ice cream in front of the TV. They are *thinking* about fitness, and that's good. But you can't think yourself fit. You have to take action.

How often do people say to themselves that someday they'll do something about it?

"Someday" usually arrives after that first coronary, or when—middle-aged, 50 pounds overweight and barely functioning outside the brain—they discover that they can do little of what they used to be able to do, and they can't find any of the youth and vigor that used to make life so sweet.

The lucky ones respond sooner. They keep hearing about quality time, but when they find time, they don't find much quality. They come home from work too tired to play with the kids or to go out to a movie. And they decide to do something about it.

For all of our scientific knowledge, medical advances and state-of-the-art information technology, more and more people are finding themselves in the condition I just described. It is just *so easy* to do nothing and eat poorly in the U.S. today! We are blessed with the fruits of profound technological innovation—things that keep our minds busy and our bodies still!

We have access to the cheapest, safest food supply in the world. Lots of it. We also have cars, drive-thrus, garage door openers, elevators, escalators, electric can openers—the list is endless. The bottom line is that we have calorie-packed, nutrition-devoid food practically jumping into our mouths, and machines that do everything except breathe for us. Maybe it's a wonder that we're as fit as we are. Fitness used to be much easier to maintain, back before snow blowers and video games and fast food.

Even worse news is that our kids are in more desperate straits. They have a little borrowed time since the vigor of youth *temporarily* overcomes all kinds of fitness sins—but we're still talking about a real time bomb. Our young people have been bombarded all their lives with commercials for eating material that I hesitate to call food. Some of the stuff is to food what a billboard is to literature. Ever read the label on a box of cereal? For most, you might as well feed your kid a candy bar for breakfast. And with the adolescent fascination for fast food, the average teenager's lunch of choice contains more grams of fat than I eat in three days.

And then there is water, the forgotten "nutrient." I can't tell you how many kids, even adults, go through the day consuming only soda pop or coffee. We'll talk later about the tremendous deficit to your health that comes from even mild dehydration.

Put all that garbage in the stomach of a generation that gets its exercise playing video games and you have a blueprint for disaster. If you think health-care costs eat up an obscene part of our national resources now, just watch the first quarter century of the millennium.

Enough doom and gloom. If you want to avoid being part of that large group of statistics, the good news is that you are in charge of your body! You can make pivotal choices now and every day for the rest of your life— it's called commitment and discipline. Each choice will take you either a step toward or a step away from being one of those health-bomb statistics.

As for your kids, well, most of us know that they have an incredible ability to tell their parents no. But like everything else you try to teach your kids, what you *do* will speak far louder than any words. Statistics show time and again that habits are handed down generation to generation. What do your kids see *you* eating? How much exercise do they see *you* getting? Are they watching you smoke? You *are* a role model, even if it doesn't often seem that way.

So this is the turning point. The preceding pages sounded the wakeup call, described a solution and started to paint a picture of how that solution might look for you. If you know you need to do something now about your health and lifestyle, then read the chapters that follow.

Part One is my story, some of which is painful and not very pretty. I fit that second, lesser-known stereotype. I'm not sure any bodybuilding champion ever emerged from a frame as fragile, malfunctioning and physically and emotionally scarred as the body I had in 1976. And my entrepreneurial career didn't start out much better.

Talking about my own adversities in this book is more about hoping that my experience can benefit others. When life turns out to be very good for someone who thought he was dealt the crummiest of hands, then he *owes* the telling of the tale. We all have adversities; many of you had your own crises growing up, whether they were physical or emotional. Hearing the story of my struggle and healing may help you experience healing, too. The biggest key in this part of the book is the tremendous power of turning a negative into a positive, regardless of the situation.

Part Two will explain why I really mean it when I say the kitchen is my most important training room. You may never get into bodybuilding—or you may already be seriously into the sport. Either way, you'll want to know why *a single can* of diet pop six days before a competition can cause me to lose the contest. You'll want to know what different foods will and won't do for you, why timing your meals is important—and lots of other information that is important to anyone who cares about his or her body.

Part Three is about sweat. Yes, we are going to talk about exercise. There is no substitute for it—whether you're pumping iron, walking, or exercising in your living room. The constant bombardment of marketing and advertising tells us to *get* things, but fitness is something you must *do*. I'll show you many different ways to do it, from designing a fitness program without spending a penny to a workout for a hard-core bodybuilder.

Part Four shows you how the mind, in the end, is your most powerful tool. Bodybuilding definitely builds muscle, but it's the mind that runs the program and even wins the medals. The three D's—devotion, determination, and discipline—are what get every ounce of achievement possible from your body.

In this book, it is my sole objective to light your fire and get you passionate about your own health. I want to show you that health and fitness go way beyond skin deep—a healthy body supports every facet of life that is important to you. I want you to learn from my experiences, to see what your true potential can be, and seize your true quality of life—without needing a life-threatening crisis to force you into it.

I have had my own experiences with near-fatal wakeup calls, and by the grace of God I listened both times. Listen to the words—"wakeup call."

That means your body has the ability to warn you when the big hand is getting ready to slap you. Don't let it slap you. Don't ignore it, don't wait until it's a closed fist and knocks you to the ground. Let my experiences pay the price for you—that's just smart business!

I personally have dug through the ruins of a health crisis, piece by excruciating piece. Some of you have, too. The greatest lesson I learned is that the human soul and body are capable of tremendous feats, far greater than most of us ever realize.

I also learned how few people know their true potential, or the key role that health and fitness play in tapping it.

If you have heard one word I said, your view of health and fitness has changed already—you know it goes far deeper than muscle and sweat and swagger. You sense an intangible something, an exciting energy bubbling inside, just beneath the surface, and you sense that it is *yours*. You are champing at the bit to get going, to try it on and try it out, even though you are not quite sure what *it* is. *It* is a deep well of energy, begging you to let it out. That energy is exactly what this book is about, and fitness is the custom-made key you can use to unlock the door.

You have now had your first taste of what I am all about. The door to a whole new health experience is open for you. You are daring to believe that it may be opening to a whole new life experience. And you are about to walk through it and see for yourself. If you walk through, and keep reading, you are already a champion.

Some of you can scarcely picture yourself as a champion. *I am talking to you.*

You are the champion of your life, whether you believe it yet or not. *You* are still that kid running carefree and strong in the summer sun. If I sparked even a glimmer of that belief in you—or even just a *desire* to believe it—then you owe it to yourself to keep reading. Forget what anyone else tells you about who you are or what you can be. Turn the page and grasp the power within you to shape and transform your life by committing to something as simple and powerful as health and fitness.

Walk with me through the following pages and open your heart to the real and amazing quality of life within your reach. If you do, I promise that your view of yourself will change, and you will see your amazing true potential to be healthy, fit, and happy. Now let's get down to the nuts and bolts of your new life.

Part One:
Scars and Barbells

I

A World Turned Inside Out

Picture Bensonhurst in the 1970s.

What's that?? Yuh dunno Bensonhurst?

Sorry. Even today I sometimes forget that Brooklyn isn't the center of the universe. It sure seemed to be when I was growing up.

I lived in my grandmother's ancient six-unit apartment building from the time my parents brought me home, brand-new, until I moved out on my own when I was 19.

The streets of Brooklyn were the whole world to me. Now, I'm not old enough that I missed the TV revolution, but we spent a lot more time on the streets than we did watching TV. So I didn't get a wide or varied view of what daily life was supposed to look like. Like most kids, I assumed the world was the same everywhere as it was in my neighborhood, in my family.

To me, the heartbeat of America was 67th Street, between 10th and 11th Avenues, right outside the building my mother's mother spent half a century paying for and where Frankie Puccio lived right across the hall. Out my door, knock on Frankie's door, and we already had a forward and a goalie for a street hockey game. And we played a *lot* of street hockey.

I don't know what your image of Brooklyn street hockey is, but if it's anything like what my friends in the Midwest have in mind these days, it's a whole different world. We may not have had ice, but we were serious about the game. We all had paper routes or we shined shoes, or both, and went out and bought genuine equipment: pads, sticks—the whole nine yards, even the nets.

Our "home court," 67th Street, was a one-way street. We'd put the hock-ey nets on rollers, set up in the middle of the street and go at it. It was an

13

unwritten rule that the cars shared the street with us. We would let traffic back up until somebody honked and yelled loud enough. Then we'd roll the nets aside, let the cars go by, and start checking, passing and shooting again.

Hockey was a big part of the fabric of our lives. Everyone wanted to master the best technique and have the best equipment to do it with. "Lifting" the puck was an essential technique for any serious hockey player, so we all went out and got plastic-tipped sticks, held them over the stove to bend them, then taught ourselves how to lift the puck. It was a street puck—solid plastic that took a lot of beating—and it would give *you* a pretty good beating if you got hit with it.

I was always the goalie, but I taught myself how to use a curved stick anyway. One day, my neighbor, Anthony Fiotto, was on his way home from Catholic school; those of us from McKinley Junior High were already out on the street playing. Anthony was standing nearby talking to a girl he was trying to impress, so I decided to impress both of them.

"Hey Tony," I yelled. "Look at this. I can lift the puck!"

So Anthony looked at me, and I laid into a slap shot. It must have been a good one because Anthony never moved. He took it on the chin and on the lip. Opened his face right up. He was standing there in his school uniform, with blood all over his face and his shirt and tie—a total disaster. And the girl he was impressing just stood there with her jaw open.

As kids, we were always getting hurt in one game or another. We were a real athletic bunch, always on the move—not on school teams, but in the neighborhood. We did have Pony League baseball, but most of the action was right there on 67th Street. Street hockey, punchball, two-hand touch football—with the sidelines running from sewer to sewer.

Our touch football games were probably rougher than if we had suited up and played on a real field. The first time I broke my nose was playing touch football. We'd mark the yard lines on 67th with chalk, and then we'd go over the lines with a candle so they wouldn't disappear in the rain.

The neighborhood seemed to take care of us, like one big family. It was an Italian neighborhood—except I was the only kid on the block without an Italian name. My father was Danish. That was all right, because my mother is as Italian as they come; I had a fine Roman nose to prove it— until it took a beating in that touch football game, and a few other times.

The private "clubs" dotting the neighborhood were colorful, to say the least. Starting at around age 9 or 10, that's where I would shine shoes for pocket money. The clientele was pretty colorful, too; along with average workers and businessmen, there were a few loan sharks, plus some serious gamblers. I suppose I shined shoes for a hit man or two. If I was lucky, I'd come home with $11 or $12 in my pocket.

There was never a dull moment. One time someone stole the jewels off the religious icons at the Regina Pacis Church on 65th Street. Neighborhood talk put their value at $2 million. That was probably a little inflated for the sake of effect, but the real issue was that they were worth more than money to the parish. The Gallo family and the Gambino family put out "word" on the street: Bring the jewels back within 24 hours, or else. No one knows who actually stole them, or what happened to the thieves, but in 24 hours the jewels were back on the statues.

So that's where I grew up: a tough, tight-knit ethnic neighborhood. And when you live in a neighborhood like that, you have to be extra tough if you happen to be small. I got involved in a lot of fights, but not because I had a chip on my shoulder. I certainly wasn't a bully; I was slim and short. Most of my girlfriends weighed a few pounds more than I did. Like a lot of things—including the illness that almost killed me—I thought it was a part of growing up. As I said earlier, my view of what was normal was totally based on what I saw around me every day. The occasional fight just seemed to go with the turf—even the fights that turned nasty.

When I was 14, I got stabbed in the shoulder. It was just another fight with a kid who was a troublemaker from the time he was in kindergarten. I don't know if I would have won the fight, but he made sure I didn't by stabbing me. I wanted to retaliate, but my Dad said: "Listen, somebody more stupid than you will take care of him someday. I'm calling you stupid for lowering yourself to his level." It took eight years, but my Dad proved to be right. My sister called one day and said the neighborhood bully who had stabbed me was now a 22-year-old corpse, shot to death in a Brooklyn hallway.

Some of what we thought was normal is definitely *not* what I want for my kids today.

Sadly, there was also a lot of well-publicized racial tension in Bensonhurst. If a black family moved into the neighborhood, a brick would go through their window—or a firebomb. Police cars got set on fire. It was part of neighborhood "reality" back then. Although the neighborhood gave me a lot, I am grateful that it evolved and eventually rejected such blatant racism. Brotherhood and equality among all human beings is extremely important to me. When I see these kinds of things now on TV, or as memories from the past, I am appalled and saddened that it once seemed just a part of "how things were."

Even in that climate of racial turmoil, there was one kid at Fort Hamilton High who was, to *all* of us, neither black nor white, but simply amazing. Basketball was never my sport, partly because of my size, but I did on occasion scrimmage with this kid. Of all the intimidating situations and people I've faced in my life, shooting hoops against Bernard King, even in an adolescent pick-up game, ranks right up there at the top of the list. And it should have, considering Bernard went on to become an NBA star and one of the best-known scorers of the 1980s. It was fascinating to see someone who was *so good* at something. We couldn't wait to see him get beyond high school, because it was so obvious that he was going to the top.

I loved grade school and junior high. I got average grades or better, came home each afternoon to load up on Twinkies and milk and jelly junk, then went out onto 67th Street for the day's urban athletics. It was the only groove I knew, and it seemed just fine.

High school was another story.

In our world, it was completely normal to live your entire life in the neighborhood. After all, it was the center of the universe, right? When I got to Fort Hamilton High, in the 10th grade, I was right on track to make it through and meld into the neighborhood as an adult. Every high school has its groups or "cliques"—the jocks, the popular crowd, the Goths, the preppies, the burnouts, and on and on. I became a "Bomber Jacket"—the nickname for those of us who wore leather bomber's jackets and wore our hair shorter than the other main group, the Hippies. We caused minor problems, but we went to class. On the surface, except for being shorter and lighter than I should have been, I was pretty much your typical Bensonhurst adolescent, up until high school, anyway. That's when my world, and my body, started to tear apart.

For starters, high school was even tougher than the streets of the neighborhood. It was not a pleasant place to be. If you wanted to find some trouble—kids smoking marijuana, kids wanting to start a fight—the place to go was the boys' room at Fort Hamilton High. And sometime in the 10th grade, I began to need ever more frequent trips to the toilet.

There is no way to tell the story of my disease without talking about trips to the toilet and about bodily functions. It's a humbling experience to do so. It's not exactly a conversation starter; maybe that's why so few people know about the disease, even though it is a potentially deadly affliction suffered by over one million Americans. Even more suffer from other diseases of the lower digestive tract. It simply is not a popular or pleasant topic, but it is one of those things that only gets worse if hidden away.

So consider this fair warning if you're reading while curled up with a bag of chips and a pop. You shouldn't be eating them anyway.

My parents thought I was just short and on the scrawny side. My friends thought I was just short and on the scrawny side. Long after I should have known better, I thought I was just short and on the scrawny side, and that I would hit my growth spurt someday. Inside, I knew something *had* to be wrong, but every teenager wants, above all else, to feel normal. So I told myself I was just naturally thin. My intestines began to tell me otherwise. I went into denial because I was just too embarrassed to tell anyone that I had diarrhea so often. The crisis started to build when other people began to notice how often I had to use the bathroom.

My mother, father, sister and I were crammed into a two-bedroom apartment with a single bathroom. Sometimes I would be in there for an hour, in distress, while an anxious line formed outside. Nothing like an audience to increase the pressure.

I lost so many half days at school that my teachers began to think I was avoiding class. At home, I started to hear: "It's Monday morning and Peter's going to have *another* excuse." In reality, I was *really* sick. At least at home, I had some privacy. At school, even if I was willing to risk excusing myself from class so I could hustle down the hall, the boys' room was a gauntlet in itself. Often I chose to stay home instead.

I adjusted, and just like many other aspects of growing up in Bensonhurst, I told myself: "Well, that's the way it is. That's the way it's going to be. That's me."

I still played street hockey or punchball every day—though I'd have to excuse myself too often. And afterward, when I should have been doing homework, I would sleep. Little cuts appeared in the skin around my eyes. I was athletic but scrawny; active but seriously fatigued. My mother often had to wake me up for dinner.

My condition put stress on our already borderline-dysfunctional family. Like so many families, there was a lot of love in our apartment, but things weren't perfect by any stretch of the imagination.

My Dad smoked—little Between the Acts cigars that left him waking up with a cough. And, after putting in a hard day at work, he drank too much. Not falling-down drunk or to the point of abusing us, but too much to go through life without it taking a serious toll on his body. In that respect, he wasn't so different from many of the other dads in the neighborhood. He was a telephone lineman who would take me on wonderful hunting trips, a solid guy whose idea of a good time was to stop at a Flatbush bar at night and bend elbows with his friends. When I was 14, he enrolled me in karate school. I wasn't too thrilled, but it was perfect for Dad because karate school was right down the street from the Avenue U Bar. A year later, he had a 15-year-old son who was a runt, and who had taken to spending an hour at a time in the bathroom. I'm sure neither of us was exactly what the other wanted him to be, but we were father and son.

My sister was struggling with her own urban adolescent problems, trying to be a young woman while sharing her room with a teenage brother.

My mother was protective of everyone, which circled back on her and sooner or later made her everybody's target. There was tension and there were shouting matches.

I internalized it all. Arguments were a good excuse to go take a nap.

Denial and reality met head-on one night that will stand forever, I hope, as the most embarrassing and frightening moment of my life.

I had saved up $900 from my paper route and shining shoes. My Dad and Mom threw in another $500, which was enough to buy a Ford Maverick, my first and favorite car. A New York learner's permit allowed me to drive at age 15. It was more likely the Maverick than my Roman nose that got me a date with a girl I had been eyeing for weeks. With my wheels, a great night at the movies and a visit to the diner, I was determined to make a first-class impression.

Something from the concession stand—popcorn, maybe, or candy—whipped my stomach like you would never believe. Driving away from the theater, with my date starting to get cozy and romantic, I was in agony and terror. I didn't know how long I was going to be able to keep control of my insides. I told her I had a flat, pulled the Maverick over to the curb, and got out.

Away from the lights, dizzy, I started hemorrhaging. I could see the red flowing down the crease of my cream-colored pants, along with the contents of my bowels.

This, finally, was something that couldn't be denied. I was a 15-year-old kid who had just turned inside out, literally and figuratively, standing alongside a curb in Bensonhurst. I was athletic, young, street-smart, and immortal. But the most vile contents of my body were drooling out onto the street.

I was in shock. *Literal* shock. And it seemed somehow logical that the thing to do was to get back inside my car. I did. My date was disgusted, and caught a cab home. I drove home, snuck into the apartment and cleaned myself up. Then I went to my mother and said: "Mom, I've got a problem."

She took me to almost two dozen doctors, where I was tested for what seemed like every known disease—diseases I thought were extinct, or only existed on other continents or in B movies. Malaria, typhoid, tuberculosis. Even leukemia. Medicine was well into the modern era in 1976, but the doctors could not figure out what was wrong with me.

One day the phone rang and a doctor told my Mom to take my temperature, "right now while you're on the phone." The thermometer registered 99 degrees, and the doctor had an "Aha!" The lab had reported mononucleosis, the temperature confirmed it. Everybody was supposed to feel relieved.

My white cell count was abnormal, that was true. I did have mono. But mono wasn't the real problem—it was only a symptom, due to lack of proper nutrition. We didn't know that, and followed the standard drill for mono treatment.

I stayed home for three weeks, took a little medication, got my immune system functioning again, and went back to school. And boom! The same old bathroom symptoms returned, along with the chills.

We went through all the tests again, including upper and lower GI's, this time with Dr. Imperato, an internist on 75th Street in Bay Ridge. Before I was through with him, this very wise man, since deceased, would not only diagnose my problem, he would tell me some of the most important things I would ever hear in my life—things I *needed* to hear about myself, and about life.

In mid-November, Dr. Imperato put me in Long Island University Hospital in Brooklyn for still more tests. I was supposed to be there for the weekend, and I was upset about it.

A normal teenage sense of immortality plus a little over-developed street macho add up to a sick kid who, even after all the trauma, after baffling the medical establishment for a month and a half, resents being sent to the hospital. I suppose it was mental self-preservation. So in I went, with a big chip on my shoulder.

When I came out nearly two months later, my entire body was about the size of that chip. And I wouldn't have to worry about going back to Fort Hamilton High again.

2

The Bridge

My health condition continued to baffle the hospital's finest doctors. At times it seemed they were grabbing for straws—and each straw was attached to a sore part of my body. The nurses were running out of places to draw blood. The lab had run almost every test they knew. My weekend in the hospital started to look more like permanent residency, and my limited adolescent patience wore thin.

Like most kids, Christmas was my favorite holiday—gifts and snow and lights. After almost a month in the hospital, I started asking if I'd be home for Christmas. And every day the doctors would come through and say: "Looks good," or, "I don't know." And they kept ordering new tests. To be honest, I wasn't sure what was more exhausting: the illness, the not knowing what caused it, or the medical procedures aimed at determining the cause.

Finally the doctors decided that exploratory surgery would be necessary. Christmas was only a couple of days away, and I wasn't scheduled until after the holiday. That meant Christmas in the hospital. Out the window I could see the snow and the lights of Brooklyn. Christmas in my family was going to happen without me. The turmoil in my head had gotten as bad as the turmoil in my abdomen.

The staff had no idea what was wrong with my body, but it was pretty clear that I had a serious attitude problem. I was holding in all of the strain of my illness, plus the impact it had on my family. It was a pretty big load for a teenager, and Christmas is when I finally "lost it."

Hospitals are an intimidating, strange place under any circumstances, but Christmastime in a hospital is downright surreal. Staff members are in the

21

holiday mood and they have their office holiday parties like anyone else. There are Christmas trees in the wards, cheerful decorations hanging from the wall—sometimes over someone who has a few hours left to live. And when the holiday itself comes, a lot of the regulars get some well-deserved time off.

I grew almost accustomed to being a sort of living lab sample, but only for my regular cast of examiners. But since I was in a University hospital, it was a teaching hospital. Doctors have to learn somewhere, and they don't learn on well people. So, around Christmas 1976, I was put on display for what to me was just a whole new group of pokers and prodders and viewers. The medical interns were in command, and I was exhausted and wary.

The curtain closed around my bed and the chief intern presented my puzzling condition (not me) to six of his colleagues. Out came the flashlights and probing fingers, and they asked each other questions as if I were either not there or couldn't hear. They wanted me to drop my hospital gown for a whole new set of strangers. One of them reached to touch me and I let loose.

"Out! Out!" I yelled. "The interview is *over!* Get the hell out!"

I'm not sure who was more in the wrong there—the doctors, or me. I know I was angry and belligerent, and I know they were polite and callous. I needed to protect what shred of dignity I had left, and they needed to do their job. One thing is sure—it gave me a deep appreciation of true bedside manner from experienced physicians.

After my outburst, I shut down emotionally and physically. The staff left me alone to cool down and didn't bother to come and take blood that night.

Dr. Imperato, the internist who had sent me to the hospital and ultimately to the surgeons, came to see me the next day, to see the kid who was still struggling to hold a chip on his shoulder, still trying to be cocky and macho—basically, still internalizing all of his turmoil and emotion. I was a pouting child with clenched fists and crossed arms.

He sat on my bed and turned my head away from the cartoons or whatever I was watching on TV.

"I want you to understand," he said. "You're a very sick kid. Two things can happen. You can either feel sorry for yourself, or you can start showing some emotions and be a human being. You can stop the denial and you can grow up."

I hated him.

I hated him for putting me in the hospital, I hated him because I thought I'd never get out. I hated him because I didn't know what else to do with all of the pain, anger and fear I was holding inside.

He went on.

"You know what your problem is? You hold everything in. It's OK to let it out. You can cry." Dr. Imperato knew what he was doing. He went on antagonizing me, "tough love" style, trying to get me to crack so I'd let it all out before I exploded. And it worked.

I finally broke down and cried, because I was scared to death. I felt trapped by my body. Something was very, very wrong with it and nobody knew what it was. Letting my feelings out didn't diagnose my problem, but it took the pressure down several notches. Getting some of that pressure off was key, because I needed all my energy to fight for my life.

The exploratory surgery did solve the mystery, if not the problem. It turned out to be more than exploratory, in fact. I left the operating room minus a foot and a half of my large intestine—plus a diagnosis. I had something called Crohn's disease. I learned that I'd had it from the day I was born and will have it until the day I die.

In a way it was a relief, finally, to have a name on which to hang all this misery. But after so much time, even the solution to the puzzle was a shock. Hundreds of thousands of people have this unheard-of disease? I have it severely enough to fade away to less than 100 pounds approaching my 16th birthday? Nobody can find it for three months and scores of tests, until they cut me open? And to find it, they literally spread my guts on an operating table? And they didn't put all of them back in?

Yes. Yes. And yes.

And to sprinkle a little more joy on the situation, they diagnosed me with lactose intolerance. That meant that unless I wanted to spend the rest of my life in the bathroom, I had to forget milk, cheese, ice cream, and—the crowning blow—*pizza.*

Double whammy. But the lactose intolerance, devastating as it was to a teenager who thought junk food and pizza were the staff of life, was nothing more than an inconvenience. And, besides, you could probably cheat occasionally, right? This Crohn's, however, was something else.

Besides losing a chunk of intestine, I came out of surgery with stitches in my rectum to close fissures that had ripped open from so much distress. I woke up wearing an ostomy bag. That's one of those lovely pouches you carry under your clothes to capture body waste. Maybe we'll be able to take it off when the torn tissue heals, the doctors said. Or maybe not. So although I was relieved to have an answer, I was far from being out of the woods.

Crohn's is a mystery in nearly all respects except what it does to the body. It attacks and ulcerates intestinal tissue in a random pattern. Weak spots can appear simultaneously from one end of the digestive tract to the other— from the esophagus to the anus—though the vast majority of Crohn's occurs in the large or small intestine. There is no known cause and no known cure, but medication and diet will help put the disease in remission. Diagnosis is touchy, because Crohn's sneaks up slowly, and because the symptoms suggest other diseases. My own symptoms would remain with me, mostly in lessening stages, for a year. And I would be on medication for four years.

After nearly two months in the hospital on IV's, which I rolled into the bathroom with me many times each day, I went home weighing 86 pounds. I struggled to get the mental picture together, to be able to say: "Well, I'm not a freak after all. They found out what it is." I still felt like a freak. The first two weeks out of the hospital were a running nightmare that worsened each night. Despite my frail body I perceived myself to be a 1,000-pound stone around my parents' necks. Mom and Dad, who mistakenly thought of Crohn's as being something like an ulcer, falsely blamed each other for causing it. Dad said Mom had stomach problems, and had passed them on to me. Mom said Dad's late-night arrivals from a night at the bar—after which they would argue—made me nervous. And I, of course, blamed myself for causing *their* bickering. Now we were truly a dysfunctional family.

Tension and stress do not cause Crohn's. But when stress is introduced to an existing Crohn's situation, it's the icing on an ugly cake. Think of yourself in the most painful gastro situation you have ever experienced—be it flu or whatever. Then imagine putting yourself under the most stress you've ever experienced. *Now* imagine what's going on in your abdomen. So it went on 67th Street, in spades.

I suspect that everyone, once or twice in his or her life, considers choosing not to live anymore. For teenagers, who haven't had the pain and privilege of seeing their way through serious adversities, the lure of suicide is amplified a hundred times. Even minor obstacles seem overwhelming. My obstacle was that I was living in a body torn up in ways I couldn't have imagined—except maybe in a 90-year-old. I was loaded with physical and emotional scar tissue, 99 percent of it on the inside. There was some real grief there—my body was not like everyone else's, and that was never going to change.

There is a fine line between grief and self-pity. The grief side is necessary. The self-pity side is optional—and it can get dangerous.

If anybody ever had more self-pity, he's the champ. I wanted people to feel sorry for me, to take care of me. And they did. Some of the neighborhood people laughed at her, but my Mom kept delivering the *Daily News* for me—in the snow—so I wouldn't lose the job. I couldn't go to school, so the school sent tutors to the house. I wanted people to be sympathetic, and I played every ace in the deck to make it happen.

But was this the way I had to live the rest of my life? With my mother babying me and going out of her way to prepare just the right foods, and my father, when he finally did get home to dinner, saying: "Oh, we have to have *this* again?" followed by me running out of the room. I began to think

I was such a hassle to my family that they would be better off without me. Thank God things came to a head before I had a chance to act that out. One night at the dinner table I took a dish of food—I don't remember what it was, just that it was steaming hot—and I threw it against the wall, shattering the plate and leaving a gooey trail down to the floor.

There was dead silence.

Then everybody started crying and babbling—and *talking*. What's going on here? Let's regroup!

We had our first really good talk. Through that talk, I realized that all the self-pity wasn't the real me, that it wasn't getting me anywhere, and that I was finished with it. It was an act, a coping mechanism, and it didn't work. I decided it was time to get my mental program in gear. It was like throwing a switch. When it happened, it was nearly instantaneous. If you drew a graph of my attitude, you would see a long curve sinking to the bottom of the page—and then a vertical line going almost straight north out of sight. Really. That's the way it played out.

After our talk, I realized that my parents were going to lead a happily married life again, despite this little obstacle who lived in the next room. I realized that the school would function without me. I realized that street hockey had not disappeared from Brooklyn in my absence. I realized that it wasn't any fun being sick. The world was going to go on, and if I didn't change, it would go on without me. I wanted to do something about it.

Once I could clearly see through the self-pity, everything Dr. Imperato had told me suddenly made sense. I could see myself with a clarity I'd never had before, like the truth was displayed before me on a mile-high movie screen. I could go into a corner and melt away and cease to exist, or I could take this handicap and turn it into a challenge. No person or thing could fix it for me or take it away. It wasn't the world against me. It was *me against me*. That was the beginning of my lifetime dedication to turning obstacles into opportunities—the beginning, as it were, of what grew into "Peter's Principles for Health, Fitness and Lifestyle."

I can't really begin to explain what happened the moment that billboard lit up, except that it was a moment, and it was very dramatic for me. It was mid-January 1977, early in the morning—it wasn't quite daylight yet. I got in my 1970 red Maverick and drove down to the waterfront. Not to take my life, but to *celebrate it*.

At the west end of Brooklyn, the Verazanno Narrows Bridge hangs across the sky. It is an awesome sight, and it is still a very special place for me. If the hard hats who create these blue-collar works of art ever once understood what they were doing—besides stringing massive coils of steel, driving rivets and making welds—this must be the once. It's the world's longest suspension bridge, a hard-hat masterpiece running from Brooklyn to Staten Island.

When I was 5 years old, Dad would take me down to the waterfront to fly a kite. The bridge towers were already up, and that summer we watched them hang the deck. I was awed by it, and it was a picture I would never forget. Its sheer size and complexity would always be sobering to me. As the years went by, it became the place I always returned to get things in perspective and sort things out—my personal reality check. If you ever get to Brooklyn, you've got to see it for yourself. Brooklyn isn't exactly a tourist destination, but you're not going to beat the view anywhere.

I could stand on the Brooklyn shore of the narrows, just above the bridge, and just a turn of my head from right to left and I'd see what seemed like the whole world go by.

Up the Hudson River lies the southern tip of Manhattan, the clutter capital of the world, 26 miles of skyscrapers and million-dollar deals and poverty and geniuses and crazy people. Turn your head and into view comes the Statue of Liberty—out in the water where the Hudson River and the East River come together—with various incidentals in the background, like New Jersey. Then, as you pan to the left, come Staten Island and this incredible bridge reaching out through the sky to touch it. Beyond the bridge you see nothing and everything—forever, the Lower Bay and on out into the Atlantic Ocean. In one turn of the head the view changes from an incredibly concentrated mass of people and money to an infinity where no one walks.

I love water. I love sunrises. I can't count the times I rode my bicycle down to look at the water in the early morning, to look at the bridge and the high-rises.

Shore Road runs along the water, and above it lie the high-rises of the Bay Ridge neighborhood. These apartments mesmerized me nearly as much as the bridge. It was the elite section of Brooklyn. The view was a lot different than from 67th Street, three blocks from where "Saturday Night Fever" was shot at the Club 2001 Odyssey. A few months later, in 1977, the whole country would be watching John Travolta and his Bensonhurst pals being drawn to the bridge.

On that crisp January morning, I took a blanket, got in the Maverick, drove down to Shore Road and waited for the sun to come up.

It must have been about 17 degrees. I parked on a hill going down to the Beltway, shivered under my blanket and watched the cars go by, and then watched the dawn rise left to right across water and the bridge and the Statue of Liberty. It may sound melodramatic, but I think there are many people who seek these moments of solitude in a place where they can be alone with their thoughts to get back on center. I thought about what a jerk I'd been lately. And I said to myself: "Damn. I want to live. I want to *live*." Something *changed* inside me that morning.

A huge weight was gone and it felt like a new fire had been lit in my heart. It was as if all of that internalized negativity and pain and hurt—all the fear that had been constricted for so long—were suddenly let loose from a catapult. I was sitting still in the old Maverick but I was moving forward at the speed of light.

I wanted to thank everybody—from my mother for delivering the papers to the doctors who poked and prodded and cut on me. I wanted to thank the school for sending tutors. I wanted to thank my Dad for showing me this bridge. It was like an Academy Award acceptance speech run amok. I thanked people who would have been shocked and bewildered if they had heard the thanks.

It's called gratitude.

I was grateful to be alive. In that moment, I realized that I had *survived*, and in that moment, I stopped being a victim. It was a turning point in my life, the most critical to this day.

I thanked God, of course. And I struck a deal. It wasn't really a prayer. It wasn't really even a *religious* moment. It was more like the guy hanging by a branch off the cliff, who suddenly has a serious talk with God. Anyway, it was a talk with God, and I struck a deal.

I told God that if He would just make me better, I would do *anything*. Make me normal and I will not get in trouble on street corners, I will not take so many things for granted, I will listen to the doctor, I will take care of myself, I will make *myself* healthy, *I will not be this cocky kid from Brooklyn.* And on and on.

It was a powerful fire that was lit out there on Shore Road, and everything that has happened to me since I can trace to the decisions I made that morning.

3

"They Look Like Toothpicks"

After my surgery, Dr. Imperato told my parents to put me on a nutritious diet and avoid milk products because of my lactose intolerance. And, by the way, this kid needs to get his body back—so you ought to get him a set of weights. There you have the glamorous start of my bodybuilding career, with me weighing in at an intimidating 86 pounds.

My father went out and bought a 110-pound set of weights for me as a belated Christmas present. It was sitting in the basement the morning I went down to the waterfront. Those weights were among the hundreds of things I thought about as the sun came up. This time, I thought about them in a completely different way.

About a year earlier, my cousin, Louis Romanzi, had taken me to Boston College for a visit. Louis played football at BC, and this was my first chance to rub elbows with some big-time athletes. I was duly impressed. When I saw all these guys in the weight room pumping iron, I thought, yeah, it would be nice to build your body into something that awesome. But I didn't feel the least inclined to put in that kind of sweat or work. It never occurred to me that bodybuilding would ever be a part of my life.

Louis wasn't just an iron-pumping football player, he was a genuine bodybuilder. When I'd visit my uncle's house in Bayshore, I'd pick up some of Louis's muscle magazines. And I'd laugh at the whole idea. This was a sport? And I'd say something like: "These guys are all either gay or they're muscleheads," which was pretty bold considering that Louis was older and at least 100 pounds heavier. I remember looking at a picture of Arnold Schwarzenegger all greased up for competition, and I said: "Why would anybody want to do that to their body?" I couldn't comprehend it.

But when my last semester started at Fort Hamilton, before I got really sick, I signed up for weight training. It was only once a week, though, and I didn't work very hard. I probably missed a few of the sessions because of illness before I left school for good and went into the hospital. I learned how to tell a barbell from a dumbbell, and a curl from a press. That was the extent of my weightlifting knowledge on January 17, 1977.

I'll never forget that date. I've become a goal-oriented person, and I write my goals down on paper. When a day goes badly, or if something gives me even a trace of self-pity, I open up a kitchen cabinet or desk drawer and there it is: a calendar with all my goals for the year, including the ones I've already achieved, neatly checked off. Try it; you'll be surprised what it will do for your perspective and focus. The very first date I ever wrote down was January 17, 1977. I was in the basement of our apartment building, and I decided to log my progress as I built my body back to what I dreamed of being above all else: normal.

The doctors at the hospital had said not to exercise for a month. But my fire was lit and I was ready. Well, actually, my physical strength was more like an ember than a fire. But the fire in my mind was ablaze. I was careful. Just a few curls and a couple of bench presses at a time. I didn't do sit-ups because of the bag on my stomach.

Despite my light little effort at exercise, my mother and grandmother would come rushing down the stairs to make sure I wasn't hurting myself. It was kind of funny; I had made these great strides forward, and didn't want or need any more babying, but I was still getting it anyway. The difference was that now it was comical instead of tragic.

I turned my life around down in that 100-year-old basement. That's a serious fact of my life. But there was a slapstick element to it all.

For starters, I could only make a space about eight feet wide. And the ceiling was low—about six feet—which meant I couldn't do any work standing up. There was dust all over the place, which didn't help my various allergies. The smell was atrocious—first because of my own sweat in a cramped and airless space, and then because I was right next to the garbage pails and the incinerator chute. I'd be counting reps, and on "six" a dead fish or such would hit bottom of the chute a couple of feet away. On the other side of the gym were the clotheslines, usually loaded with sheets and underwear. And people were always walking through, going to the clotheslines or to the garbage cans.

Welcome to the original Peter Nielsen's Total Fitness Club. I should have had business cards printed. Down at the bottom they'd proclaim: "Unmatched Ambience."

About two months after coming home from the hospital, I went back.

The doctors took the bag off my stomach. I cannot tell you what it meant to a 15-year-old for this particular roll of the dice to come up a winner. It meant, most basically, that on my 16th birthday—March 16, 1977—I would be performing a basic bodily function normally, the way I assumed every other 16-year-old in the universe performed it. Clearly, somebody was answering those promises I made on Shore Road. In later years, speaking around the country to raise money for research into Crohn's and other intestinal diseases, I would come into contact with scores of people who are leading normal, productive, happy lives without the luxury of reversing that roll of the dice. It's just one of the thousands of ways I have learned that whatever your circumstance, others have it worse.

Fueled by my new degree of freedom, I became even more of a terror with my 110-pound set of weights. I added another few iron plates and picked up some dumbbells. By the time I was finished with my grand-mother's basement, I had almost a thousand dollars worth of equipment.

Those were fun times. The tutors came to our apartment, and in the end I graduated six months ahead of everybody else. I basically had nothing to do but study and bring my body back. I started alone, and then Frankie Puccio—my hockey-playing friend from across the hall—joined me. And then Tommy Lupo from 64th Street. We were three oddball musketeers, pumping iron amid the fish carcasses and the drying underwear from 3C. Once, one of us pushed some iron a little too high and snapped a plumb-ing pipe. Now we had the only gym in town with a water hazard.

In the beginning, I worked with a little supermarket book that showed how to do different exercises. Then I started to wonder about this whole *bodybuilding* thing. I had to be impressed with Lou Ferrigno. He was almost from the neighborhood, growing up two miles away on 64th Street, and he was a Mr. Universe—soon to be immortalized on TV as "The Incredible Hulk," the green guy with all those muscles. I kept buying exercise books, soaking up new material like a sponge.

I learned so much in that basement, not just about working out, but about life and reality. Years later I would own a gym with half a million dollars' worth of equipment, but some of my best workouts were in that basement gym. Name-brand shorts and engineered fabrics are great, but the body gets just as fit working out in a cotton T-shirt and no-name shorts. Fancy gloves? Calluses work just fine for me. Never once as the years went on did I get impressed or taken in by pricey paraphernalia, because it didn't mean a thing in my basement gym. All that mattered was that burning desire to get better. If you've got that fire—my version of it or your version of it—the other stuff is just that: stuff.

My buddies and I improvised workouts like jazz musicians. Once again, we took what was there and made it into something better. For example, the basement was full of bricks. We turned them into a platform for back exercises, or would place them so our feet would have more of a stretch when we lay down. Outside in the courtyard, when the weather got warmer, the fence gate did double duty as a brace for dips, and a tree became a support for stretching exercises, plus it offered a nice sturdy branch for pull-ups.

The point is, not having a fancy health club membership is no obstacle (or excuse!) if you want to work out. If you can't afford it, or if you just don't want to work out in public, no problem. Do you have a *chair* in your house? A rope? A towel? All these things can be excellent pieces of exercise equipment. It's too easy to get focused on the place, the equipment, the *stuff*. What's more important is to focus on *you*.

In the basement, I pursued my self-education in exercise. Upstairs in the apartment, I was launching my education in nutrition. Right from the start, I made myself a human guinea pig. Besides, no one else seemed to have a great deal of information about my condition.

Let's see, today's subject is lactose intolerance. Let's try some pizza. OK, stomach all torn up, off to the bathroom. Experiment complete. Thesis confirmed: you play, you pay. It became clear that food was either nutrition or poison for my body.

I had a lot to learn in the area of nutrition, and I was really on my own with it. The doctors saved my life, but nutrition was not their specialty. And the mystery of Crohn's, particularly in a teenage patient, had them looking to *me* for answers. Like a well-conducted science experiment, I carefully documented my nutrition and the effects it had on my body, on my Crohn's. I'd get a call from the doctor, and he'd ask: "Peter, what happened that time you indulged and ate several slices of pizza?" And I'd say: "Well, doctor, the first two slices weren't bad ... " They would document the information and, I hope, used it to benefit other patients as well.

I took vitamins and I tried protein powders. I read everything I could find on the subject of nutrition because I had to rebuild my health, and my body rejected so much of the junk I used to call food. The real dietary tricks of preparing for a bodybuilding competition would come later. But very quickly I found myself well-versed in basic, sound nutrition. I learned what proteins and carbohydrates and fats mean to your body, where they go and what they do when they get there. I put myself on a dietary regimen that at first was merely an exercise in discipline, but which I soon learned was an exercise in health. In other words, I started to feel better.

All in all, the self-pitying kid who had wanted to strike out at a very wise doctor was coming out of his shell. These were exciting times.

These were also scary times.

Not long after leaving the hospital, my blood count was still wrong. The mono had returned and I had to fight if off again. I learned to be patient with my recovery and to recognize that setbacks are not the end of the world.

About a month after having the ostomy bag removed, I returned to the hospital for a scope test that would check all of the repair work on my "plumbing." The doctors found cancerous polyps on my colon, totally unrelated to the Crohn's. The polyps were tiny, and the doctors were able to scrape them off with no trouble. But they were cancer nonetheless, and they scared the hell out of me.

I'm not sure what would have happened if I had heard the word "malignant" when I was in the hospital at Christmas. Two months later, it was certainly no picnic, but it gave me an *opportunity* to see how far my attitude had come. It was the fruit of my newfound discipline and turn-negatives-to-positives policy—practicing it each and every day for just a few months was like a survival insurance policy. I wasn't really conscious of it at the moment, but my new attitude gave me a mental steadiness that played right through that ordeal. It was the beginning of a lifelong lesson: Crises will come in life; the key is to be prepared. So I had set out along my little obstacle course—you know, life—with a completely different head on my shoulders and working toward a new body. Not many days after the doctors scraped away the polyps, I was back down among the garbage pails pumping iron.

I reached a healthy plateau down there with my slowly growing collection of weights—and my radio. Music was very important to me. I played guitar and sang in a neighborhood garage band that we put together back in the sixth grade. Our first "public appearance" was at a block party where we conned the hired band into letting us sit in for one song. These four rockin' little kids gave the older guys a real run for their money, and a career of sorts was launched. We played Bensonhurst parties and weddings for almost a decade. My sister joined the band too, playing tambourine and singing. I still wonder how far we would have taken it with that band if I hadn't been nudged down the path of health and fitness. Probably not much further than the neighborhood—my series of broken noses gave me a pretty unique intonation!

The music on my radio was the background to a steady, pleasant groove: work out in the basement, meet with the tutors, study, work out in the basement, pore over anything I could find to read about nutrition and exercise, experiment in the kitchen, work out in the basement. After spending so much time sick and distressed, my only focus was to get well, and I made the most of it.

I had never before known what it was like to feel good.

The Crohn's had always been there, just waiting to come full-blown out of remission. That happened when I was 15. It could have happened when I was 6 or 60. But from toddling age onward I had been a sickly kid. I was a short kid because I wasn't getting proper nourishment—the Crohn's was stealing almost all of it. Every birthday I would get a fever and chills because anxiety—even though it doesn't *cause* Crohn's—can work with the disease to trigger gastro problems. So I was a thin, short, quick-to-tire kid who got sick whenever something made him nervous. My parents say that whole syndrome started back when I was 3 years old. Finally getting well and putting some musculature on my body was an indescribable high. I started to feel *normal*.

In January 1978, a year and a month after my Crohn's surgery, I became a certified, mid-year, home-tutored graduate of Fort Hamilton High School. I was well on the way to putting my disease into remission, still the proud owner of a 1970 Maverick, and no longer looking anorexic. By mid-summer of 1978 I was probably a whopping 145 pounds or so. I felt like Hercules. I wasn't about to wander too far from this health and fitness lifestyle because it was the only thing that could give me the healthy, normal life I craved.

It was never my intention to set foot in a real gym. But all the magazines said that if you wanted to make genuine progress, you had to be in a competitive environment with somebody a little better pushing you. Primed to take the next step in my new life, I started to think about finding a gym.

Meantime, a friend of my mother's told me about a guy in Flatbush. "He trains champions," she said. "You ought to check him out."

So I did.

The guy in Flatbush was Julie Levine, chiropractor by trade, powerlifter by avocation. When I walked in his door he stood about 5-foot-10, and carried a very compact 200 pounds or so.

The name of his place was R&J Health Studios—on Avenue U between East 27th and East 28th streets. It was the Mecca of East Coast bodybuilding, though I didn't understand the first thing about that. I just knew this was where Lou Ferrigno had trained, and that Julie had been Ferrigno's manager. Ferrigno was at his peak then—really hot. If you didn't know about Ferrigno, then you probably weren't alive—and you definitely weren't in Brooklyn. But I didn't know the first thing about Julie. I tossed my fears aside and went.

I introduced myself and Julie said: "Hiya kid, howya doin'? Looks like ya been training your arms a couple years. What happened to your legs? They look like toothpicks."

Ouch. Welcome to the gym.

I was devastated. Hurt. Embarrassed for my basement gym and the bricks and the garbage cans and ... what was a runt like me doing there anyway? I was about to turn on my heel and walk out, but then my pilot light kicked on, and my attitude squared itself back up. You know what? My legs *did* look like toothpicks. But he also said I looked like I'd been working out *a couple of years!*

Adversity really *had* become my best friend.

Of course, under my breath, I called Julie every profane name I knew. And then I paid him $178 for a year's membership. In a long and strong relationship, it was the only time Julie ever charged me for using R&J's facilities. But I'm not sure it was the only time I called him names under my breath for telling me the truth!

Mecca of bodybuilders or not, moving up to Julie's was not like moving from the basement to a plush-carpeted suburban health spa. At R&J, if you didn't smell the sweat, you didn't have a nose. It was quite famous, but not fancy, and definitely not chic. It had character—and characters. My ragged attire fit right in, and so did I.

Walking down the stairs you had to watch yourself, because pieces of the steps were missing. The dumbbells were the big old round Charles Atlas type, with chips knocked out by too many collisions with the floor. Frequent eyeball calibrations were necessary: "Let's see, this is an 85-pounder, but with that chunk gone it's probably about 79." Julie was big on people, not on stuff.

So R&J wasn't fancy, wasn't in a wealthy section of Brooklyn, and there wasn't a lot of pretense among the clientele. They were there to pump iron. The customers—ranging in age from the teens to the 70s—just wanted to be the best that they could be. Basically they were vulgar, full of lies about their romantic conquests of the previous evening, and not particularly interested in where the Dow Jones Industrial Average was going that afternoon. It was a social club with the aroma of exercise. It was wonderful.

Julie presided like a revered bartender. R&J wasn't a health *salon,* it was a health *saloon*—like a good neighborhood bar you'd start hanging out in at 20 and stay until you died, as long as that same guy was standing there with the towel and the talk. If he dies, the bar dies.

I was 17 years old, training at Julie's place and surrounded by bodybuilders. I was full of myself because my body and I had fought the Crohn's into remission. I started thinking about the future, about what part this bodybuilding thing would play in it. I had to see how far I could take this thing. So I slipped out of town to enter my first bodybuilding contest. It was Mr. Armstrong County, a teenage amateur competition somewhere in

Pennsylvania. My father drove eight hours to get us there. I finished fifth.

I remember sleeping in the back seat, stretched out with my trophy. I could still see the expression on the face of the person who won the contest, and I knew that I really wanted to do this thing—and I wanted to finish first, at least once. R&J would be the place where I could make that happen. I had made it 90 percent of the way down in Grandma's basement, but the very tough remaining 10 percent needed Julie and the gym.

I decided to go for it. First I went to work on my "toothpicks." At home I zeroed in on nutrition. At Julie's I zeroed in on my legs. I used Julie's comment to fuel me—I decided I was going to show this wiseguy what I could do. And I did. I added nine inches to my thighs.

That's taking a negative and making it a positive.

In my next competition, Mr. Teenage Appalachia, I won my class and finished second overall. I had to laugh when my biggest criticism came from the judge who actually said I looked freakish—he said my legs were *too big*.

4

Trophy Time

That chilly sunrise monologue out on Shore Road lingered in my mind like deathbed testimony. I felt like I was on trial, having promised the moon in return for becoming a normal kid. So I became a gym rat with all the dedication of an avowed monk. If Julie's gym was a seminary, however, it was by a good stretch of the imagination. It held its own sort of purity, though, for those who wanted to get focused on bodybuilding.

I began to fantasize how far I might get in this newly discovered world of bodybuilding. It was an irresistible fantasy—a quantum leap—from a feeble, rotting, dying body to solid muscle, vibrant health and a growing rack of trophies. I had the audacity to say to myself, *Why not?* Lou Ferrigno had gotten his start at Julie's. I bet I could do it, too. When I was sure no mind readers were nearby, I dared to think: "Someday, people will say: 'This is where Peter Nielsen worked out.'"

Nobody worked harder.

Julie said he learned a lot about me from the way I responded to his wisecrack about my legs. "You can't say things like that to certain people," Julie said. "But I knew you could take it." I'm not sure if he really knew that or not—he was just lucky my specialty was taking negative feedback and making it fuel for my fire to get better. And I was just plain lucky that I stumbled onto Julie.

It also turned out I was lucky to have had those karate lessons I hated so much. I had dreaded the ride to Flatbush every single time my Dad took me to class. Some kids get dragged to piano lessons; some get dragged to dance lessons; I got dragged to karate. I think I earned my brown belt fueled purely by the animosity I built up on the ride to class. By the time I got there, I was ready to crush everybody in the place because I despised being there so much. Karate just wasn't in my heart, but I did find a way to reap some special benefits from it later on.

I realized that karate had introduced me to discipline and self-esteem. It taught me coordination and a little grace—basically how to choreograph my body and to have better timing. The agility it gave me increased my confidence—even when dancing with the opposite sex. When I began competitive bodybuilding, I reached back to those dreaded karate sessions to improve my stage posing the same way Arnold Schwarzenegger had used ballet lessons. Most bodybuilders get a least a little grief from their friends or family, especially about posing on a stage. I'm sure posing on a stage doesn't sound particularly macho to most people, but posing is just a fancy word for flexing every muscle group in your body while simultaneously presenting them for harsh evaluation by a set of critical judges. It takes a lot of guts and a lot of grace to put all of your most personal work on display like that; it's also an incredible rush to take home a trophy for it.

Almost from the beginning, I had an affinity for posing. That's good, because it's a major part of competition. If I wanted to win, I couldn't look like I'd rather be somewhere else. Something about the pain and scars of my illness made me thrive on the soul-baring that goes with being up on stage all alone. It wasn't how well I could swing a bat or how much gold I could wearing around my neck—I was the product. It was my way of showing just how good I could be on a physical level. It was also a statement about me as a person, because getting to that level of physical development meant I took what God gave me—which at the time, didn't seem like much—and then applied every bit of discipline, dedication, sweat and nutritional wisdom that I could pull together. It was much more than physical development. Maybe it was because my physical being had dwindled almost to nothing, and putting its reconstructed polar opposite on display was a testimony of how far I'd come.

I had to learn to "strike a pose" and get "cut"—get that ultra high muscular definition a competitor has to develop just before competition. That meant I had to face any insecurity about my body head-on. It all brought a sense of pride, freedom and achievement that I had never experienced before.

Julie really put me on track for competition performance. In 1979, he first got me posing in front of a mirror almost every day—not for vanity, but for progress checks. He showed me how to use the mirror to check my muscle development, and to tailor my exercise regimen for body symmetry, which is a key competition factor. He taught me to see self-examination as part of the craft.

Trophies are won and lost based on what the judges see. If I wanted to improve what they saw, I had to learn to use the mirror to evaluate what all those curls and presses and dips were doing for my body, and where to make adjustments.

We started taking all this seriously not long after the Teenage Appalachia contest. It seemed like the contests were always far away, but my Dad drove me to all of them. In 1979, I became a teenage bodybuilding terror, winning one contest after another. Once I won two contests in a single weekend. My training was together, my diet was together, and it was all paying off. Life was good.

And of course there was a girl, Yvonne Wind. She lived near the gym, taking care of her emphysematic father, and we started dating soon after I first met Julie. Yvonne was wise beyond her years, and she truly was the wind beneath my wings. Sunrise promises on Shore Road or not, I'm not sure I would have taken this bodybuilding thing so far without Yvonne.

She'd cook dinner for me, make sure I got over to Julie's even if I wasn't in the mood, sit down and learn about nutrition with me, and encourage me. Even cocky street kids thrive on encouragement. After I won my first contest, Yvonne made it seem like I was on the cover of *Sports Illustrated* when I really wasn't anywhere except on Julie's bulletin board. Her belief in me made a big difference in my life. It was one of those rare teenage romances that really meant something.

My Dad—who at first regarded bodybuilding as weirdness from deep left field—began to see that it was good for me. He even got caught up a little in the competitiveness. When the weekend came, we'd hop in the car and go pick up another trophy. But a total, full-time commitment to the sport was something else. To Dad, that was still *deep* left field.

I was totally committed to it. Except for making a few bucks doing odd-job construction work, my only work was on my body and my mind. Both kept getting stronger, and the trophies started piling up. By standard measurements of success, however, I had become your basic well-proportioned dropout.

In 1980, when I was still 19, Dad cut a lot of red tape and wined and dined his boss to get me my first and only "legitimate" nine-to-five job—as a lineman's assistant for New York Bell, following in his footsteps, making decent money, enjoying full health-care coverage. This was the real world and this was a job to be prized. The streets were full of people who would kill for a job as a lineman's assistant. So off I went into the "real" world.

The first doorbell I rang was to make a disconnect for nonpayment in Bedford-Stuyvesant. A heavyset woman with a less-than-pleasant disposition answered the door and people started screaming in the hallway. I put my screwdriver up to remove a phone jack and a gang of roaches came crawling out of the wall. Then a very large man emerged from a bedroom and joined in the shouting. Out back, where I had to disconnect and test some other wires, a group of very tough-looking guys were playing cards. I finished the job and got in the truck.

I turned to my partner and told him, "No amount of money is worth this."

Ten days later, I quit. I went to my boss and told him I was sorry. He said: "Don't worry. Your Dad is going to take this a lot worse than I am."

He was right.

My father didn't understand the dreams that were forming in my mind, and looking back, I know it was hard for him to see. All he knew was that I had come out of the hospital three years earlier as a sick kid and was doing OK—but devoting all my time to lifting weights and counting grams of protein and fat. And now I was spitting on a job that he had used to raise a family. All he saw in the gym was ego. He didn't fully understand the will to survive that had led me to the gym, or the mental discipline and personal dedication it had taught me. He didn't share my vision of the future: that pumping iron might lead me to a world of achievement. And I was still a few years away from the maturity one needs to understand the difference between making something an important *part* of your life and making it your *whole* life. I'm sure it wasn't the first time a father and son just couldn't see eye to eye. I guess this was your classic clash of the generations.

Anyway, my father quit talking to me.

By that point, Julie Levine had realized that this kid from Bensonhurst possessed an extraordinary level of determination. He devoted still more time to my physical program and to jawing with me about what it takes to be a champion. I was on track for the Eastern Teenage America, by far my most serious competition yet, and Julie was getting on track with me.

That's when I knew I had the opportunity of a lifetime. I was learning everything from gym etiquette to kinesiology from the master himself. One thing Julie preached was not to take things too seriously, not to lose perspective. I was young. Some of Julie's lessons I absorbed better than others.

One day Julie took me to see a doctor of sports medicine who worked with bodybuilders. He gave Julie an honest assessment, the way a horse trainer might analyze the conformation of a thoroughbred. Not while I was in the room, of course.

Genetics can give a bodybuilder a handicap or a head start. Just as you won't see too many 6-foot-10, 290-pound figure skaters, you won't see champion bodybuilders with ultra-high calves or biceps, or with long legs beneath a short torso. This is the sort of thing the sports doctor was evaluating for Julie.

A few weeks later I got the message secondhand when I overheard Julie talking to somebody else about it. The doctor's diagnosis? Peter will become a local champion, possibly a state champion. If he's tremendously lucky, he'll become a regional champion. As far as a national champion, he'd put his license against it.

More wood for the fire! If negatives were the raw material I used to build my positive outlook, I was definitely a rich kid. I'm sure Julie didn't intend for me to hear that conversation, but it was a good thing I did. You can lift a lot of barbells and skip a lot of junk food with words like that ringing in your ears.

All of the contests so far had been teenage amateur events. The Eastern America show was an important one, however. It was at Lincoln Center, and it seemed like half of Brooklyn made the trip into Manhattan. My Mom was there, Julie was there, half of his clientele was there, and if things got dull we could have put my old street hockey team together in 30 seconds.

If you've ever seen a bodybuilding competition, you know the finals are where things get really hot. Most of the serious judging is done in the afternoon, away from the crowds, the same as compulsories in figure skating. The afternoon scene can be like going into a college gym and stumbling onto a hard-fought game in some minor sport. The players and officials are intent, all right, but not much is happening otherwise. Then at night, when the finals of a bodybuilding competition occur, the scene changes dramatically.

There's a crowd, music, spotlights and an exuberant emcee. Every contestant has his own entourage of sorts, his own loyal followers, cheering wildly for or against each competitor. In this contest, if a bodybuilder happened to be from Brooklyn, the cheering was likely to be a bit more colorful than if he was from, say, White Plains. Posing in front of that crowd was very long way from the solitude and privacy of a mirror at R&J Health Studios.

Lincoln Center was also a long way from Pennsylvania and New Jersey and some of the other outposts Dad had taken me to win various local competitions. This uptown contest was wild and scary—and I loved it. I won my height classification, I won best in every body part, I won overall. I wish I had a transcript of what the announcer read that night, with all my Bensonhurst friends stomping and whistling. He said something about a young man who had overcome adversity and was on his way up the ladder, and he said: "We have a special presenter to give Peter his trophy as Mr. Eastern Teenage America—Pete Nielsen, Peter's father."

Whatever this thing was that his kid had gotten into, Pete Nielsen had decided that it must be important. I wasn't an opera singer or an actor or a politician, but I was on the stage at Lincoln Center collecting a trophy. And my father, who hadn't talked to me in six weeks, was handing it to me.

We both got teary-eyed. And Dad was with me for the rest of the run to the top.

He started carrying my posed picture in his wallet, and a glossy of me went up on the wall at the Avenue U Bar. That was a definite first in *that* bar. Dad also forgave me for dumping the lineman's assistant job and helped get me put on-call for construction work, mainly handling a jack-hammer on road crews. He had a son with a real job, and I had a father who supported my dream. Julie canceled my membership fee at R&J and gave me a key so I could work out at 4 a.m. or midnight or whenever it fit my schedule. Life became a crazy pattern of tooth-rattling jackhammer work on weekdays and competitions on weekends. I wore a hard hat and I wore a bikini, I worked under traffic lights and I worked under stage lights, I crunched pavement and I consumed protein. It was an interesting mix—I've yet to meet anyone else who passed through the late teen years and into young adulthood along quite the same career path.

I was definitely the oddball among the construction crew. I was the only construction worker, for instance, who ordered vegetable omelets made with no yolks. If you're not used to them, egg-white omelets do look pale, but they still taste great. All that's taken out is the cholesterol and fat. I was never able to talk the guys into it, and they were never able to talk me into a pile of greasy bacon and eggs.

Those construction crews usually decided I wasn't wrapped too tight. It may have had something to do with the day I did a number on a taxi driver. To start with, it seemed like every time I ever worked on a jackhammer it was either 100 degrees in the shade or minus-10. On the day in question, it was so cold I was shaking *before* I picked up my hammer. I worked under a little framed tent that was supposed to cut wind chill; I was rattling and hammering and chipping and shivering right in the center lane. A cabbie pulled up, laid on his horn and just sat there, braying away. Only a New York cab driver would sit in traffic and honk his horn at a tent.

I was cold and miserable and the honking did not help. In a second, the cabbie wasn't irritated—he was so scared he nearly relieved himself in the fare box. My body was in pretty good shape by then, so I cradled this 70-pound jackhammer like it was an Uzi, raised my left arm in the air like I was leading a charge on enemy lines and came running out of the tent pulling the trigger, Rambo-style. I will never forget the look in that cabbie's eyes! He got the point. He stopped blowing his horn. My co-workers just rolled their eyes.

Mixed in with that silliness was some true craziness. One morning at about 4 a.m., I was just turning the key at R&J for an early morning work-out. A guy came walking out of the restaurant next door, saying goodbye to everybody. He couldn't have been more than six feet away from me as I unlocked the door. A car pulled up to the curb and suddenly—pow, pow, pow—a gun was fired. The man next to me fell to the sidewalk with parts of his head missing. The car pulled slowly away.

Like I said, it was an interesting lifestyle for a teenager. Never a dull moment in the big city.

In Bensonhurst, everybody was crammed together. The streets were full of people. Life was fast-paced and *a la carte*—there was a store for everything. When I moved to Michigan, somebody picked up a phone and said: "Let's get a pizza." It was the funniest thing I ever heard. In Brooklyn, nobody gets *a* pizza. You get a *slice* of pizza. And you fold it and eat on the run, whether you're wearing warm-ups or a three-piece suit. When I was a kid in Brooklyn, you bought your slice at the pizza parlor, your bread at the bakery (but bagels at the bagel shop).

I even had a friend who worked at a *pork* shop. Five zillion cuts of meat and sausages, but not an ounce of beef or chicken or fish in sight. My friend once said: "Peter, I'm working out but I'm still flabby." And I told him: "I think you ought to find a new job."

With everybody out on the street, playing hockey or hustling a buck or getting to work or running between the bakery and the pork shop, Brooklyn was just as different from suburbia as it was from a farm in Kansas. On a hot summer day, strolling down the sidewalk wearing a T-shirt, anybody who spent a lot of time in the gym stood out like a red popcorn kernel in a bag of white.

Back in the neighborhood, we had a name for somebody who was what we thought was a cool, macho dude—he was a "coozhine" (say coo-ZHEEN). John Travolta's character in "Saturday Night Fever" was a coozhine, for those of you that remember. It was a look, an attitude, and every city and small town has its own similar brand of cool. Bodybuilding was most definitely a good way to be a coozhine in Brooklyn.

One very unique thing about Brooklyn was its bodybuilding culture—it had a history of great bodybuilders. It's like jazz musicians. Why are such an overwhelming percentage of the truly great jazz players from certain cities? Well, that's a complicated question. But one reason is that a lot of jazz musicians grew up in a culture that attached some importance to the music, gave it some respect. If you wanted to go down to your basement and play scales for 10 hours a day, that was OK, because that's what it takes to become a truly great jazz musician. That's the musician's sweat equity. Sometimes you'd have a basement, or a neighborhood, that produced an amazing number of great jazz musicians. Among bodybuilders, Brooklyn was such a neighborhood. And R&J was the best basement of all.

I kept the promises I made, and my body was responding. I was healthy. I was also collecting more trophies than anybody. After turning around the hardship and illness, you bet it was fun being a coozhine.

5

Muscle Glitz

I dreamed of having my own apartment in Bay Ridge, overlooking the narrows and that incredible panorama that had mesmerized me since childhood. My parents were supportive. Needless to say, my sister was supportive—my freedom would mean freedom for her in our tiny apartment.

My parents told me: "Save up before you move up; get yourself a job and sign a lease." Very reasonable advice, the kind that parents give. My response? "Hey! I've got a month's rent. I've got a security deposit. I'm goal-oriented. Who cares if I don't have a regular job?"

I'm not sure it occurred to me that I also didn't have any furniture.

I knew just the place I wanted. I moved in shortly after flunking out as a telephone lineman's assistant. I wrestled the jackhammer and made the rent. But I still spent a lot of time on 67th Street, because some of the finest Italian cooking you'll ever find was still upstairs in my Mom's kitchen.

At night, though, I rested my head in Bay Ridge. I could do my running along Shore Road. I had an *elite* address, which at the time seemed important. The sunrise was free every day, and the water and the bridge came with it.

It was September 1980, and I was 19. From then through the fall of 1984 I would win another 60 bodybuilding trophies. I would suffer two serious relapses of Crohn's. I would pose in Times Square and have my picture in *Newsweek* and *The National Enquirer* and I would appear on "Good Morning, America." I would go to Central America to win my biggest title, and I would make personal appearances on several continents. I would make some decent money. I'm very proud of those achievements, but the picture was never quite as rosy as it should have been.

For one thing, I was surrounded by dry rot in the form of anabolic steroids. In the early '80s I think it would have been fair to lift an eyebrow at nearly any athlete of tremendous bulk and Adonis proportions. In the '88 Olympics, the Ben Johnson saga proved that you didn't have to be a lumbering football lineman to enhance your performance with steroids. My sport, bodybuilding, was awash in steroids.

There are two statements I can make unequivocally, with God as my witness: First, I never used anabolic steroids. Second, I came so close that I get sick thinking about it.

It was everywhere.

There was a kid up the street from me who was using steroids and bragging about it, even showing syringes to his friends. One day he started passing blood in his urine and got rushed to the hospital. I knew another steroid user who dropped dead of a heart attack in the gym, where he was supposed to be getting healthy.

The most insidious part of the steroid epidemic, in fact, was that the biggest advocates were the athletes themselves. They played Russian roulette with their lives, satisfied when the results of their liver function tests were way above normal—but just below the point of internal bleeding. One kid told me he would be willing to take steroids even if he knew it would kill him, as long as he could win Mr. Teenage America first. A lot of sickness was running around wearing the trappings of fitness.

The pressure to try steroids was immense, particularly in the teen years—when the mind lacks maturity and the muscles have trouble achieving size. Many competitors regarded me as a candy-ass for not being a user. I'm sure that others believed that I was a user and was a candy-ass for lying about it.

One of the dozens and dozens of times another weightlifter pushed anabolic steroids on me in the gym, I bought some. Dynabol. It was my first or second year of working out.

I was young and susceptible. But instead of opening the bottle and tearing right in, I took it home and stashed it in the bathroom. I don't know if wisdom, ethics, common sense—all the things that insist no human being ever ingest steroids—would have prevailed. I like to think so. But in the end, it was two things—my goal-setting nature and Crohn's disease—that assured I did not take the lunatic path.

Remember my calendar? I actually wrote down for a Monday: Start Dynabol. Meanwhile, I would think about it. Thanks to the Crohn's, I didn't have to think too long. I started bleeding internally, with no help whatsoever from anabolic steroids.

Whatever teen fantasy I might have developed about bottled muscles died instantly. I nearly screamed out loud: "What am I *doing?*" I flushed the steroids down the toilet and went into a cold sweat.

Was I so vulnerable that I could forget why I started lifting weights in the first place? How could I so carefully choose and measure the fuel I put in my body at the dinner table, and then even think about gulping this poison? The stuff isn't even a narcotic and its pull is that strong. Incredible.

Later, I would go on stage in competitions and discover that the guy on my left and the guy on my right were both pumping steroids as well as iron. I would discover that some bodybuilders I had thought to be natural (drug-free), were not. A frustrating, contradictory, mentally debilitating knowledge revealed itself over the next four years: Bodybuilding is a great sport that should earn much wider participation and media interest, but it was hopelessly corrupted by a deadly genie in a drug bottle.

Today I spend a fair amount of time talking to kids about the danger of drugs—any drugs. I hope my talks do some good. I hold my body up as an example of what they can do "clean and natural" with their own bodies. Any effort to get the anti-drug message across is good. "Say no" is a great message—without that other word in front of it. "*Just* say no" misses the point. If it were a case of *just* saying no, there would be no problem. Whatever things kids do wrong, it isn't because it's the *hard* thing to do. It's because it's the *easy* thing to do.

The other cloud over my rosy four years of glory was in my own head. I stayed close and true to my Shore Road promises about my body, but it would take a while before I really stopped being that cocky kid from Brooklyn. Glory is a tough thing for a young person to handle. Pretty soon I wasn't just a coozhine from Brooklyn—I was *uptown!* I put bodybuilding and the glitz and the glamour ahead of everything, and did some incredibly stupid things with my personal life. You might say I suffered from progressive muscle-headedness.

I dumped Yvonne, for one thing. And, toward the end of this four-year run, I tried to be a party animal while simultaneously keeping my body in top form. Too many times I met myself in the morning coming from tinseltown to the gym. I thought I could handle it, but it just can't be done. Maybe for a quick minute when a person is young, and that's it. I was young, and I used my quick minute to the max.

I also spent a lot of money. That's not a sin, and it doesn't affect training, but it was awfully stupid.

Mixed in with that relative insanity, I did make some choice good moves—pretty gutsy ones, when I look back on it.

In 1981, for example, I had had just about enough of hanging onto that jackhammer. It seemed to me that if I could spend my weekends striking a pose on stage and collecting all that silverware for my effort, then there ought to be a way to make a buck at it during the week.

What I did was audacious.

It went something like this: Let's see, this is the greatest country in the world, so I should go into business. What have I got to sell? Well, I've got a physique and some clips from the muscle magazines and the *Daily News* and I've got a real talent for posing. Where can I sell that? Well ... how about Studio 54? This was back in the day when Studio 54 was *the* nightclub in New York—in America—to be and be seen in.

I was like a 20-year-old bomber pilot in World War II. I didn't know I couldn't do it so I did it. I grabbed my portfolio, took off, and dropped it on the desk of Studio 54's managers.

"Listen," I said, pointing to the clips. "This is me. I've won best poser in every single one of my contests."

"Great," said the general manager. "So what?"

Well, as I said, music has always been important to me, and I used it in my bodybuilding routine, almost like choreography. But I knew I needed something a little more if I was going to be the first bodybuilder hired to work the country's most famous disco. So I improvised.

"If I had some smoke," I ventured, "and some synchronized explosions during the routine—maybe wore a dinner jacket and went through a whole act ... "

Mr. 54 was hooked. "Yeah," he said. "Continue."

I could make it much more dramatized than during a competition, where you can't use smoke. I would have some glitter on that dinner jacket, and I'd drink a potion and give the illusion that I was *changing* ...

And I said: "Well, for that I would usually get $500. But if you hire me two days a week, I'll do it for $300 a shot."

Sold.

The first night was a Thursday, a private birthday bash for Charo, who wound up coochee-coocheeing out of her own cake. But the opening act was Peter Nielsen, Mr. Whatever My Latest Title Was. The music was "Sirus" and "Super Nature." Suddenly the house lights were gone, the spots came on, all the smoke started rising and I was onstage at Studio 54. It was a major success.

That may raise an eyebrow or two, but I saw that jackhammer disappearing from my life in the rear-view mirror. Still, $600 a week wasn't all that much in a very shaky, temporary business—so off I went to talk to the proprietor at a club called Magique.

It was at First Avenue and 61st Street in Manhattan, and it was very much in vogue. Frank Sinatra had a drink or two in the club. My first approach was to the bouncer, who said: "You gotta be kidding; get to the back of the line."

The next morning I called the owner and pretended to be my own agent—Johnny Giganti or something like that—and got an appointment.

My posing career, about five minutes old, was now bringing in $1,400 a week for three nights' work.

I bought a used Mercedes. I would drop by the family apartment with all this money and my mother would get nervous. She didn't really understand—or maybe didn't believe—where it came from, and I don't blame her. I would ask my father (who figured I would be a dead-broke gym rat when I quit the phone company): "Hey, Dad. You need any cash this week?" Ouch. I'll never forget when he looked at that Mercedes. He turned to me and said: "I don't believe it. You're out of control."

He was right. But I had to learn the hard way.

There was one positive in this run of glitz that Dad didn't understand, one that would help me find a real life when the run was over. My father thought I was making money with my body, but I was also making money using my brain. I didn't have the only physique on the Eastern Seaboard. I was just the only one who put it in a package and marketed it to the glamour crowd. I had some vision and some creativity—and an entrepreneurial bent.

Julie, my mentor and friend, understood. He had given me all the training and experience I needed. He could have kept me under his wing and had a New York local hero working out of R&J. But, like the true second father that he was, he told me: "Peter, you can do even better if you go to Dan Lurie." And that's where he sent me.

Dan Lurie was a New York weight-training equipment manufacturer and the publisher of *Muscle Training Illustrated*. He agreed to meet me, saw that I had potential and put me in the centerfold of his magazine. He got me on the "Joe Franklin Show" and "Good Morning, America," and had me write a column called "Nielsen's Ratings." Now I wasn't just a kid hyping himself into the spotlight at Studio 54. The exposure Dan got for me was big-time and national.

I had saved some money from my posing jobs, but with all the publicity Dan generated, it got even better. I posed around the country and made a few appearances abroad. I got my second Mercedes. I went to a lot of parties and met celebrities like Kareem Abdul-Jabbar and Diana Ross and other A-listers who sipped cocktails and nibbled on expensive appetizers on that scene. That, of course, led to more personal appearances.

The jackhammer was long gone. But, in a way, I never escaped that unreal night-and-day flip-flop between two worlds. I still commuted between two incompatible addresses: a world of sweat, nutrition and hard work, and a world of cocktails and hors d'oeuvres and hype. I had a growing sensation of whiplash.

What I did *right* was to go, with Dan Lurie's help, to Belize, in Central America, and win the 1984-85 Mr. International Universe title. I reaped the cash rewards, began to sink even deeper into the night-and-day morass, and ultimately realized that my father was absolutely right. I was out of control. And my sport was out of control with steroids.

I had promises to keep. And it was getting difficult. So I announced that I would never compete again as long as I had to square off against bottled bodies.

"Get a life," they said. So I did.

6

New Life in Motown

Southeastern Michigan isn't exactly the wilderness. Not with a few million people, urban sprawl, the car companies, major league teams in all four big-time spectator sports and a central city with all the usual problems. It's the fifth-largest TV market, which may be the best way of summing up a town in a couch-potato world. For me, in 1984, Detroit's most important demographic was something it had in common with Pittsburgh and San Francisco and Dallas and Winnemucca, Nevada. *It wasn't New York.* When I had a chance to do a few personal appearances in suburban Detroit, Motown looked like as good a place as any to go into withdrawal from the Big Apple. I was only 23, but it was already eight years since I had dedicated my life—as best as a frightened teenager can dedicate a life—to health. And I wasn't feeling very healthy. I wanted to get away from all the temptations, to get squarely back on track.

My family and friends and everything familiar were in New York. But so were all the things that kept tugging me, as my Dad said, out of control. I had become a creature of excess—too many parties, too many girls, too much sipping Grand Marnier between training sessions, too much time using the weights for recovery instead of for training. I was a kid with his hand constantly in the cookie jar, an overgrown coozhine with his picture in the paper. For me, living in New York was like a drunk pitching his tent outside a distillery.

By comparison, Detroit is so laid back that I keep expecting to see the Beach Boys walk by. I moved in, got three phone numbers, a beeper and an agent. Shortly thereafter I added an attorney and an accountant, and my appointment book started filling with tiny print. I was still super busy, I still had obligations, and I was taking the usual risks of being an entrepreneur. But that crazy, frantic edge to every minute of every day doesn't exist in the Detroit metro area, and I didn't miss that part of New York a bit. I adjusted quickly to my new environment. If I could eat pizza, I'd order a whole pie instead of a slice. And I'd eat it sitting down instead of on the run.

I freed my body in Julie's gym. In Michigan, I freed my mind. Unfortunately, it took more than a change of address. In fact, the early going in Michigan was worse than anything I have ever experienced— except, of course, the Crohn's. That's because I came here with a body by Fisher but with an attitude by Studio 54.

What do you suppose the Brooklyn kid bought to cruise the streets of Motown? Right. Of course. A Porsche 928, black, with several thousand dollars' worth of performance extras and a Blaupunkt sound system that put a rock band's bass player right in the passenger seat. Ego on wheels. It seemed exactly what Mr. International Universe ought to be driving. Coincidentally, the price was almost identical to Mr. International Universe's bank account. My arrival in Detroit was like Dumbo stepping off the circus train.

And what did Mr. International Universe get himself involved in? Right. Of course. A relationship with a woman who enjoyed the good life but wasn't seriously interested in a guy whose income consisted of an occasional personal appearance fee and a small endorsement contract. I might have been a minor celebrity in New York and in the world of bodybuilding, but in Detroit I was lucky to have a part-time gig pitching fruit juice. It was a struggle to put gas in the Porsche, let alone foot the bill for wining and dining a girlfriend who had champagne taste.

I suppose all those Spaniards who came to Middle America looking for gold, only to find buffalo chips and tall grass, must have had a similar reaction. Within a few months, Brooklyn was beckoning. And it was starting to look good again. I could go back to Julie's, where somebody once broke a plate-glass window and took nothing out of the place except one of my posters. (They *were* finally saying: "This is where Peter Nielsen worked out.") I could put on one of my Guinea T's, as they called the tank tops we Italians—even the half Danish ones—wore, and I could stroll big-time down Avenue U. No matter how bad things got, I could always run over to 67th Street and get the finest homemade spaghetti dinner in New York. The temptation was huge; not for the glitz, but for the comforts of *home.*

The girlfriend had turned out to be, at least from my own point of view, my most serious relationship since Yvonne. It was more serious because I was older. But with Yvonne it had been unconditional. This time it wasn't. She wanted a lot more than I could give, and wasn't afraid to tell me so.

She could cut me to the quick with just a few words. One day she opened the refrigerator in my apartment and made a statement that changed my life. Really, it did. If you get seriously into this business of changing negatives to positives, you can find inspiration in the damnedest places.

What she said was: "You want a *commitment* from me? When you can't even make enough money to keep orange juice in the refrigerator?"

She told me I was *just* a bodybuilder—a hunk—and that I'd never make it as an entrepreneur, that she spent more cash on clothes annually than I made in a year, that I ought to go back to Brooklyn and "live happily ever after." In that instant, the very last thing I wanted to do was put on a Guinea T and stroll Avenue U.

If Julie's remark about my "toothpick" legs had stoked my fire, this woman was tossing gunpowder into a furnace. I was hurt. It brought tears to my eyes. But in the blink of an eye my vision cleared and that pain turned to purpose.

"You know something," I said, "I *am* going to become successful. You're going to turn on the television and see me. You're going to pick up the newspaper and see me. You're going to see my name in lights so bright that when you go down the road you're going to have to take a detour."

Just a *little* cocky. But as much as it stung, I almost needed her slap to wake me up, because I got focused again like never before.

I was insecure, to say the least, but I was determined to make something happen instead of retreating to Brooklyn. I was only 23 years old, however, and this was the real world. The days of Studio 54 and Magique were several years, 700 miles and a bucket of reality away. No quick tricks, no smoke and mirrors.

Every day I went to the gym and left a lot of mental garbage there—proving, as ever, that pumping iron is good for a lot more than filling out a T-shirt. I made a few bucks as I developed a personal training clientele, not just with the weights but also with nutrition counseling and motivation. I began to understand more fully that by devoting my life to practicing and studying health and fitness, I had acquired knowledge worth passing on to other people.

In the fitness world, PT means personal training. In the medical world, it means physical therapy. I was developing expertise in both versions of PT. I'm not a registered physical therapist, let alone an MD, but since age 15 I've had an obvious special affinity for people who are trying to make frail bodies better, who because of illness or accident or years of sedentary life do not fit your standard stereotype of a bodybuilder. I paid special attention to that part of my PT work, bringing out whatever percentage of improvement can be gained in bodies inflicted by lupus or arthritis, and various other diseases. And, since personal training is not something that everybody can afford, I began seeing a lot of the sour fruits of affluence—smart, successful achievers whose lifestyle took care of business but left their bodies frail and flabby and destined for intensive care. My dedication to fitness was expanding outward from my own frame toward helping others. It was starting to come full circle. I kept myself in shape, and I walked what I talked nutritionally, but I never gave a thought to the juiced-up world of competitive bodybuilding.

I had plenty of motivation to keep seeking the spotlight in other ways. For one thing, I enjoyed it. Let's face it, I grew up playing street hockey in Brooklyn and then wound up getting drum-rolled onto stages around the world. That had a certain appeal. And blame youth and a bruised ego, but I still wanted to keep my promise to put myself in lights, onto videotape and into print to prove something to the woman who had told me, in essence, that I was a dumb street kid with nice muscles. I really milked that one for lot of energy. There was also the non-trivial matter of earning a living; all those trophies and a certain amount of fame were my most marketable assets. Finally, and most importantly, it began to dawn on me that my main purpose in life is to promote health and fitness. I certainly could not do that by retreating quietly to a darkened corner.

So I launched my campaign to become a successful entrepreneur on the unfamiliar turf of Detroit, Michigan; to become known and to use my brain to do something smart with all those muscles—something that could be useful to others.

One of the first things I learned is that you can't drive a Porsche 928 on the slushy streets of Detroit in the winter. So I found an old $500 rust-buster Cadillac. I put on my best suit and my best head and drove around town knocking on doors. Ninety-nine percent of them closed right off the bat: "That's great, Peter, you're a good-looking kid and you've got a lot of ambition and a lot of enthusiasm. But not today. Come back when you can show me a track record."

It became a steady refrain. But I did my PT, I did my personal appearances for the fruit juice company, I scuffled and knocked on doors and I hung in there. And I got my balance back.

Then one night my sister called to tell me that our Dad was dead.

He had died, at peace, in the old apartment on 67th Street. Emphysema had left him too weak to fight back against a variety of illnesses. Pete Nielsen, the old New York Bell lineman, the macho father who took his son fishing and hunting, but who became enthusiastic mentor and mascot for a teenager who traipsed around the East Coast collecting trophies in a bikini, was gone.

I was so very sad and so very angry.

I loved this man who had once given me a simple little plaque with our family name on it, saying it was all he had to pass on to me, and that he knew I wouldn't dishonor it. He was full of life, yet he had drained it from himself with the garbage he put in his lungs and in his stomach.

How could I think such a thing? How could I *not?* How could he have done this to my sister, to my Mom, to me? How could I be blaming him for dying? What good can possibly come from this?

The first flight to New York wasn't until the following morning, so I had a sleepless night ahead of me. In the middle of the night I went to the gym and had the most strenuous, awkward, bizarre workout of my life, and the only tearful one. So often my workouts had helped me put everything in order, but this was a tough one. I attacked the weights with the same fervor that I wish my Dad had used to repair his health before it was too late. It was the only workout I've ever "dedicated" to someone else; if I'd been a painter, I'd have done a canvas.

We buried my Dad on Long Island. I committed to my Mom and sister to serve as the head of the household, and that in times of financial need I would be there. And I flew back to Detroit with yet another pressing motive for making a successful career for myself.

My father reached out to help me one last time when he died. There was life insurance, and my mother saw to it that part of it came to me. I was determined to roll it over into a successful enterprise, to make good for my family, and maybe show a few people that Peter Nielsen could use his brains as well as his biceps. There was enough money that I could show some earnestness to investors and carry out my plan.

My plan was simple: to combine my training talents with the medical community, to open a sports medicine/physical therapy facility where the doctors could practice and I could help people my way. Instead of throwing money into the wind as I had with my International Universe profits, I would put together something that would be worthwhile, lasting and lucrative. I produced about $6,000 for blueprints, and a few thousand for other preparations. I found three investors and committed $150,000 to landlords, construction people, equipment vendors—and signed more documents than I had ever seen in my life. I was about to enter the entrepreneurial world with the same enthusiasm, but at considerably more depth, than the day I dropped in at Studio 54. The day before Thanksgiving I was getting ready to fly back to Brooklyn for a celebration when one of my investors called:

"Peter, you know that $20,000 check I gave you?"

"Yeah ... "

"Well, it's going to bounce."

Have a nice holiday.

Investors back out of deals all the time. Finding that out was not a great consolation. Thanksgiving in Brooklyn was a day for heavy thought, and about as close as I ever came to giving up all the dreams. Instead, I went back to Detroit for a meeting with a friend who was going to try to put another partnership together.

This is where I met Charlie Baughman, who became one of the most important influences of my life. He became virtually my second father and turned my world around. You will have noticed by now that several people turned my world around at critical points—from Dr. Imperato to Julie Levine right on to Charlie Baughman. It wasn't a coincidence—some people are graced by more good fortune than others, and I have had more than my share. But I believe that *much* good fortune comes from putting your eye on the prize and going for it. There are lots of platitudes about the virtues of hard work, but simply put, nobody but a burglar or a salesman is going to find you sitting on your couch. If you're out there scouting, you'll find opportunity. Even then, too many people sidestep it instead of meeting it head-on, because it scares them.

Anyway, my persistence led me to Charlie Baughman, a former Ford Motor executive running his own company who—more than anybody— led me into the business world.

"What a day, kid," he said at that first meeting, "I've got to solve all these problems. Wait until you get older. You don't know how lucky you are right now."

"You only think you have problems, Mr. Baughman," I said, "I have to raise $75,000 in 10 days or my business plan is going down the tubes and I'm gonna be $150,000 in debt."

I didn't say it as a whine. I was just leaving the office where we'd met, and I almost said it kiddingly, to commiserate with him on his own bad day. Charlie motioned me back and said: "Tell me about it."

So Charlie learned the whole sad story of the investors who took a hike from my plans for a clinic. He asked me to lunch the next day and we talked for two hours. He decided that I was wet behind the ears, but that I was a diamond in the rough and had just met a lot of the wrong people. I had also met some of the right people, like the accountant who was carrying me on the books even though I couldn't pay the bill—and was therefore able to supply the detailed prospectus that Charlie wanted to see.

He was impressed. "You've got the makings of a pretty good team, Peter," he said. "I'm going to see if I can get you a loan."

There was another lunch, this time with two bankers. Charlie told me to wear a suit, and I was sweating into it profusely as the questions flowed over the appetizers. Then Charlie said: "Before we eat, why don't we let Peter relax a little." One of the bankers put an envelope on a dish in front of me. It contained a check, made out to me, for $75,000.

"All you have to do is sign this," the banker said. "Mr. Baughman signed the rest of the papers. He guaranteed the note."

I won't suggest that hard work and commitment are going to put $75,000 on a plate in front of you tomorrow. But I *will* suggest that there are some very nice people out there, and if a you're willing to do your homework, make a plan, get up off the couch and persist, you're liable to meet some of them. Charlie became not only a business partner but also a mentor who taught me more business savvy in six months than I had learned in my life to date. Between my penchant for turning adversity into opportunity and Charlie's financial and educational investment, we put together a first-class team: me, Charlie, my accountant and my attorney.

The clinic happened. It almost doesn't matter that after three years I was out of it, at a loss, in what amounted to a hostile takeover by the MDs. I already had opened my first Fitness Center—despite my own fears of overextending—because Charlie said: "Hey, all these people that get better at the clinic are going to need a place to work out, right?" That first Fitness Center turned out to be a major success. I recently sold it, and—following my own ideas of how a good gym should be equipped and operated— opened a Personal Training Club, as well as a full-scale Fitness Center. There is incredible power in having someone believe in you.

Other enterprises, all aimed at helping me become an effective spokesman for fitness, began to sprout all around me—dozens of opportunities to become an effective spokesman for fitness and a healthy lifestyle.

I eat, sleep and breathe fitness. I probably say: "I walk what I talk" more often than I should, but it's key to my effectiveness in helping others, especially since I talk a lot—appearances for the National Foundation for Ileitis and Colitis (now the National Crohn's and Colitis Foundation); speeches to school groups about drugs and about fitness; motivational talks to business groups. Once I spoke at a meeting of MDs who were definitely skeptical about hearing an anecdotal message from an at-home graduate of Fort Hamilton High. But by the end of my talk, many were waiting to thank me for reminding them that—though they were the experts on medicine—the holistic approach is the path toward health. I never give quite the same talk twice and I never use notes. I find out what makes each audience different and I try to reach them the best way I know how. Everybody tells me it works.

Despite that macho promise I made standing beside an empty refrigerator, my picture has never appeared on a billboard, and I'm not aware of my name in lights blinding anybody. But I began to find my mug in a Detroit newspaper quite often as its health writer, and in several fitness magazines. I wrote a book for kids, called *Growing Up Strong*. WDIV-TV, the NBC affiliate in Detroit, hired me for a fitness segment on their morning newscast. It has been fun—and useful, I think, because seldom do I talk about weightlifting. I'm more likely to talk about getting the most out of lawn mowing or (this is Detroit, remember) shoveling snow.

A few years ago I launched the Peter Nielsen brand of vitamins and supplements, a quality product packaged to my specifications, but which wasn't going anywhere. Charlie said: "Let's put it on TV, with an 800 number." Next thing I knew I was on one of those cable infomercials and sales zoomed.

Besides, I met Cindy at the ad agency that did the commercial. She became the most important member of my team, the one who is with me day and night. No one would have been more amazed than chocolate-loving Cindy that first day at the ad agency if someone had told her that very shortly she would be into a new lifestyle, designing interiors and ads for my fitness centers, broiling chicken twice a day, doing PT herself, and putting on a bikini to pose with me on the cover of a national muscle magazine. Motown has been good to me in a thousand ways, but none as great as Cindy.

And at last, I had gotten a steady handle on keeping my priorities firmly in order.

It would be fair to say that the only blinding lights anybody has to be concerned about are the ones shining in my own eyes. I got some great opportunities to share my message as a motivational speaker. I'm the first guy I know from 67th Street to publish a book. Not to worry about the blinding lights, though. I've learned that sometimes things pan out and sometimes they fizzle. But the most important things stay steady and true—like discipline, honesty, humility, generosity, fitness and gratitude. I've become, in the words of one pastor who made an impression on me: "evenly yoked." Family, career, self-worth, the worth of others—all represent a slice of my outlook, and I try to give them all my full attention. Fitness and health are the harness that reaches from everybody's yoke to the load they're pulling, and that's where I want to make an impact.

In much of the rest of this book we'll be talking about the nuts and bolts of fitness. But it's vital that you not overlook the grand design, the master blueprint. Sure, it's key to know how to perform certain exercises or how many grams of fat are in your lunch. But beneath all of that, it has to do with a healthy attitude. It's about an understanding that the body you live in is temporary housing, that it's yours for maybe eight decades if you're fortunate, and that the quality of life for you and those you love will largely be determined by how much you invest in upkeep. The beauty part is that it doesn't cost a cent of cash.

That's why I've taken up all this space telling you my own story. I want you to learn something not just about physical fitness, but also about yourself. By telling my own story, I'm putting a mirror in front of you so you can see not Peter Nielsen, but yourself—and maybe some other people you love. I don't want you to see a bodybuilder's musculature in the mirror; I just want you to see a reflection of the best you can be. I want you to see someone who is getting the most out of life, someone whose day is a series of events met with energy rather than fatigue, someone for whom *all* time is quality time.

How does the story of a Brooklyn kid with a strange disease who wound up flexing his muscles under a spotlight relate to *every* reader, as I'm convinced it does?

Most importantly, I've learned one big lesson. Life is a place where we all make mistakes. Even if we make fewer than our share of mistakes, fate will toss some obstacles and crises in our way. The greatest thing about life is that if the mistake isn't too costly, we can keep trying until we get it right. If the obstacle isn't too big, we can keep trying until we get past it. If we live well and respond fast in a crisis, we can get through it. The mistakes that millions of Americans make with their bodies are far too costly to correct years down the road. You cannot daily pour junk into your stomach, alcohol into your veins, smoke into your lungs and your butt onto the couch and then expect to make a minor course correction somewhere down the line. My life, and this book, is dedicated to helping you stop making mistakes so costly that they'll kill you, and to putting you on a *lifetime* course correction.

You don't need—nobody *needs*—a body that is as fine-tuned as mine. It's what I do for a living. It would be too much work for most people. But all of the same principles apply at a level that is *achievable* and *sustainable* for any person who wants to be fit and healthy. What I do with nutrition, exercise and mental outlook, I take to a healthy extreme. They can all be adapted to a healthy lifestyle even if your primary focus is selling stocks or hanging drywall or arguing cases before juries or raising a family. Whatever your focus, fitness will sharpen the picture.

So that focus, that attitude, is an integral part of my message. It's so important that before we get in to the nuts and bolts of nutrition, I want to spend a minute on just that—*attitude*.

7

Attitude—The Key That Turns Every Lock

It's all about health, fitness and lifestyle. In this attitude, I have found a key that turns every lock, enhances every situation in my life and puts me on the best possible path to negotiate life. It's far more than muscles and aerobic capacity and bodyfat percentages.

It's about wanting the very best health for yourself and the one and only vehicle that will carry you through your life. The good habits, self-discipline and emotional balance required to achieve glowing health will permeate every facet of a person's life.

As I worked my way from a hospital bed to Julie's gym to championship stages to a fitness career in Detroit, I learned over and over, ever more deeply, that I couldn't have a healthy and fit body unless I had a healthy and fit life. So for me, it's no small message when I say that it's about health, fitness and lifestyle. Now that message is the theme of my syndicated television program by the same name: "Peter's Principles for Health, Fitness and Lifestyle."

The lesson that I have continued to learn, that I can still trace back to that turning point at the Verazzano Narrows Bridge, is that health and fitness serve not just my body, but also my whole self, my whole soul. Sure, fitness makes the body good to look at; it also gives it the best possible chance to avoid and fight disease. But the key that turns every lock is the mental toughness that the lifestyle cultivates. I'm not talking about tough like Clint Eastwood or Xena. I'm talking about the toughness you need to make the right decision at the dinner table, every time you choose between the TV and a workout, *every* time you choose to do the right thing. That toughness starts to spill over into other aspects of your life, like deciding not to retaliate against some road-raged driver to deciding to be a positive influence instead of a complainer. It builds on itself, and it pays off tenfold during those moments of truth—during crisis. It ensures that not only is the body in the best possible shape to respond, but so is the mind.

Consistent healthy living is like making investments in a mental fortitude account.

A fit attitude and mental toughness help us to be resilient to those unavoidable setbacks we all experience. Setbacks are a part of progress, and I've had my share. Some have been recent, some I recall vividly from early in my career.

I remember being sick, somewhere around age 20. I was at the family apartment—the nest I often returned to when things weren't right. I remember being upstairs, and a friend had stopped by for a visit. I developed cramps that were so bad I thought I'd need an ambulance. My mother wanted me to go to the corner store to get something for dinner, and there I sat with that old terror and denial descending on me all over again.

In a panic, I asked myself: "How could this be happening?" I had already won a major teenage bodybuilding championship. I thought I "had my health back." You know, *for good*. I had been feeling great. And there I was, terrified all over again that I couldn't hold my bowels long enough to get to the corner and back. Was I so fragile that even after all that work I could suddenly, without warning, fall apart? I had to really take an honest look at my habits and lifestyle, and there were some contributing factors.

The bottom line was that I had been taking my health for granted again—not really watching what I ate, thinking that if a body looks great on the outside everything must be great on the inside. Common (expensive) mistake. Meanwhile, I was also breaking up with a girlfriend, and just to spice it up a little, a car I liked a lot had just been stolen—and now I was having a relapse. The lesson? Taking my health for granted is a temptation I can't afford. It can cost me everything.

It's tough to toe the line at that age; cockiness is just part of growing up, part of finding one's independence from the family, I guess. Unfortunately for me, it was far more of a luxury than I could afford, when it came to my health. It was a hard time, but I got back on my feet fast.

Around that time a song called "Eye of the Tiger" was getting a lot of airtime. The lyrics talked about how quickly we can change, how easy it is to trade passion for glory—to focus on the rewards of doing the right thing, forgetting about the right thing itself. (The name of the band was Survivor, to add a poetic touch). It also talked about getting back on your feet and getting back out there after a fall. I really took that message to heart as a young man trying to keep his priorities straight, and that song meant a great deal to me for many years. Much of my life so far had been devoted to learning that lesson. I like to think that by now I've learned it fairly well.

Crohn's was always a great reminder. I've had four major setbacks in 20 years; three were in the first 10 years, and only one in the last 10. Each time, I thought I had "arrived"—that the disease was in permanent remission. And each time nature reminded me that life is short, the path is tricky, and there are no guarantees. I gradually learned not to take things for granted, and to be mentally prepared for anything—as the saying goes, hope for the best, but prepare for the worst. Thankfully, I learned a little bit more from that mistake every time. Because of the Crohn's, I am much less able to wander off the straight and narrow because the repercussions are so costly.

Another particularly ill-timed "curve ball" took place 13 days before I got on a plane to Belize to win the biggest title I'd competed for so far, at that time. It seemingly came out of nowhere—BOOM—like somebody cut me off at the knees. This time I was heavily into training, eating exactly the right foods—and still here comes the Crohn's. Unbelievable! I remember looking at myself in the mirror, slapping myself in the face and saying: "There's no way you can get sick." Guess again. I calmed down, but I was not in the best of health when I won that competition. The lesson was that crises will happen regardless of who we are and what we want, and we have to be prepared to face them head-on.

This is why I talk about mistakes, obstacles and crises. You can correct mistakes in your life. You can fight obstacles and manage crises, but you can't prevent them. Taking care of yourself, developing the most positive mental outlook and the healthiest lifestyle possible is *no guarantee* that you won't be hit by a debilitating disease or some other crisis. Only God knows that. You could get hit by a bus tomorrow. But I can guarantee you that the right lifestyle and attitude will help you prevent the predictable ones, and sometimes vastly improve the outcome of the unavoidable ones. At the very least, a healthy mental attitude will help counteract denial and other destructive responses to a crisis.

I had read the recipe for good living, and I was following instructions, and still I got hit again. But the investment I had been making for years in my body and mind paid off, and I weathered the storm.

Sometimes the biggest risk we deal with during a setback or a crisis is the temptation to sink into self-pity. We'll get into that in detail in the very last chapter, but it was important to emphasize once again, before we launch into the nuts and bolts of nutrition, the profound importance of attitude on progress and health.

That song I referred to earlier also talked about having a fire inside, a burning desire to make it. I developed that fire because I was blessed with adversity and because I followed through on the commitment I made to get well. Being sick gave me tremendous desire to be well. It motivated me to learn how the body works, how to use it and what to put in it. I work out. I eat well. I have confidence. And because I look good, I have even more confidence. It's a total package: priorities, values, self-love, love for others, health, fitness—and they all feed on each other, one piece supporting another. And that's the whole point.

My most important message is this: There are many components to that total package, but nobody can have the *whole package* unless fitness is part of the picture. *Anybody* can find that fire within themselves and become that whole package. You just start by doing the best you can, one day at a time, for the body you're going to have to live in 24 hours a day, cradle to grave. That commitment never ends, no matter how fit you get. When we come back to my story at the end of the book, we'll see just how true that is.

Now let's get started on the first block of the foundation: nutrition.

Part Two:
Nutrition: Where It All Begins

8

Going Against the Flow

When I was growing up, the neighborhood *a la carte* pork store in Bensonhurst was a perfect symbol for the disaster area otherwise known as America's eating habits. No offense to my friend Louis, whose family runs a *fine* pork store, but just one look at the crowd lined up along the sidewalk on a Friday afternoon is enough to choke your arteries—and send you off to the Big and Tall shop to buy new clothes.

Delicacy lies in the eye of the beholder. Here are some of the delicacies for which the good citizens of Brooklyn take a number, get in line and jostle their way forward to animal-fat heaven: prosciutto, spicy ham marbled with golf-ball-sized circles of fat. Sausages, in dozens of sizes and flavors, all guaranteed to heat up dripping with fat. Brajole, a concoction consisting of fat wrapped in fat—a jelly roll of pork and mozzarella. Amazing. The mind, and the taste buds, can be trained to favor almost any kind of food—even when large, sustained doses of it will slow you down, balloon your bodyfat and maybe kill you. And that's what we grew up eating.

They call America the Melting Pot. Nutritionally speaking, it's more like the Rendering Pot. We take the *worst* nutrition of our various cultures and share it with one another. Not just the Italians, but all the sausage-making cultures offer up their cholesterol-stuffed tubes. The French taught us how to take a perfectly nutritious meal and drown it in dairy fat. The Mexicans taught us how to find vegetable protein in a mixture of corn and beans, but then they wrecked the recipe by refrying the beans in lard. Together, we savor every greasy variation, right down to the cross-cultural common denominator: the burger with fries. The advent of fast food and drive-thrus ushered in a whole new era of effortless, fatty eating.

Americans' attitudes toward food have changed quite a bit since then. We've been through just about every imaginable up and down when it comes to the prevailing wisdom about food. While some things stuck and some didn't, the '70s and '80s definitely changed our attitudes toward fatty meats and fried foods. The relationship between heart disease, obesity and a diet very high in saturated fats was clearly established and became common knowledge (not that everyone pays attention to it.) So the government recommended a low-fat diet that is high in dense, starchy carbohydrates.

So why have we as a nation continued to grow fatter and less fit? As we get into the details of nutrition, we'll see how "low fat" isn't the only mantra you need for sound nutrition, to stay fit and to maintain proper body fat. An excess of super-dense, starchy carbohydrates will make you just as fat and unhealthy as the pork shop. Think about it—what do we feed cattle to fatten them up? Fat? No. We feed them starchy, dense grain.

America has the cheapest, safest supply of food in the world—especially the sugary, fatty, starchy stuff. And on top of our excesses of starchy stuff, we pile on tons of refined sugar, soda pop, cheeseburgers and french fries.

We are the richest country in the world. But we have the poorest eating habits. We have perfected high technology and we have free public education. But we eat like illiterates. We have the money and the time to be the healthiest people in the world. But we are perhaps the least fit of all nations.

We face a health-care crisis, with medical bills eating up a disastrous and growing portion of our wealth. Many Americans have become used to the throwaway mentality of modern society; they treat their bodies like they treat their cars, ignoring preventive maintenance and care—grumbling and complaining when they have to send the junker car to the scrap yard and buy a new one. We are not so lucky with our bodies. Despite all of the advances of modern medicine and surgery, we have discovered too late that often the best repair is a poor imitation of the original. And "replacement parts" are a last resort that doesn't always work.

We spend billions of dollars trying to repair bodies destroyed by sugar, junk food, fast food, fatty food, alcohol, cigarettes and lack of exercise—and still we can't *begin* to fix the damage. We never will, really, no matter how many more billions we spend on coronary bypasses and cancer surgeries.

The incredible irony is that we could slash this suffocating repair bill by spending *less* money on junk to put in our stomachs. Who would be surprised at the repair bill for a 100,000-mile car that has never been properly maintained? Where's the surprise if the mechanic, after using up $1,000 or more of your hard-earned money, still can't get your junker running right?

That's just looking at it in terms of dollars and cents. How we *feel*, how much quality we get out of each day, can't be measured on the bottom line. Or can it? Studies suggest that trillions of dollars in productivity are lost to poor nutrition and other unhealthy habits that leave us run down, unalert and uninterested.

Who's to blame? Every out-of-shape individual, of course, whether he or she is carrying around visible flab or whether it's hidden in clogged arteries. It's true that nobody puts a gun to your head and forces you to spend $2 for a big bag containing two cents' worth of potatoes and three cents' worth of oil. Nobody forces those chips down your throat while you sit and watch TV. Well, at least not exactly. Powerful forces do aid and abet this nutritional felony, and it doesn't hurt to be aware of them. It's necessary, in fact, to be conscious of all the temptation and sugar-coated garbage that gets shoved at you day and night in modern America. Otherwise, you'll eat it.

First of all, eating poorly is easy to do in America. It's cheap, it's fast and it often tastes good. For all of our societal and technical advances, we are busier and more stressed out than ever. Picking up a sack of burgers or a bucket of fried chicken is a very tempting solution at the end of a hectic day. Doing the wrong thing is *so* much easier than doing the right thing.

Second, add in the power of cultural influence, our various heritages of fatty food. Of course, every culture has its share of healthy foods, too. But remember, we're affluent; so we take the healthiest part of our heritage's diet, shrink it down, and super-size the part that was once the smallest, most expensive part. We goop butter, cream sauce and cheese on top of perfectly healthy vegetables. We've quadrupled the traditional serving size of pasta and doubled the traditional portion size of most meals. Americans can afford it, so we choose the "reward" foods—the ones we're supposed to have only on rare occasion—almost every time we eat. Then we double the portion size! From my own heritage, I can assure you that Alfredo sauce was not something the peasants ladled on their pasta every night. Even pizza picked up 50 percent of its calories only after it was Americanized.

Third, chances are excellent that you were raised by parents who were not exactly nutritional role models. Nutrition is a modern, evolving science. Only a few decades ago, researchers were missing important pieces of the puzzle. The world of processed, packaged, sodium-laden, nutrient-robbed, sugary or greasy food was a done deal before nutritional knowledge caught up with it. Some families are into a second generation that has no idea what it means to eat fresh produce—or even to sit down together for a home-cooked meal.

Fourth, we're approaching the seventh decade of commercial television. In my day, it was Fred Flintstone selling cocoa-choco-whatevers to wide-eyed 5-year-olds who were developing permanent lifetime eating habits. It may not be Fred Flintstone anymore, but there is no shortage of cool characters pushing your kids into eating a sugary heap for breakfast. Basketball stars that—as the commercials make perfectly clear—developed their ability to jump into the sky by drinking soda pop. Role models of every stripe have sold their names, but they may really be selling the health of those kids, whose present and future eating habits are heavily influenced by the commercials. Is that a far-out, left-field viewpoint? I don't think so. The commercial messages must work, or the junk-food conglomerates wouldn't spend millions to produce them.

Finally, the educational system—meaning the schools, the household environment and the media—has not done its part to erase nutritional ignorance. Schools everywhere serve tons of french fries, nachos, cookies, and cakes—with a side of protein and vegetable. Milk is only an option, as school after school installs pop machines in the halls. We still have millions of people walking around who think that a monstrous chunk of meat in one two-ton meal is the way to "get your protein," or that a couple of Pop Tarts is a good breakfast. We are a nation that eats most of its food out of packaging that misleads or tells outright lies. Most of us don't know how to read the fine print—and even the fine print doesn't tell the whole story.

That sounds pretty grim. But the answers to a couple of obvious questions about nutrition should paint a brighter picture for you, if you're truly interested in cleaning up your act.

So who do you trust?

You trust yourself. You learn how to make intelligent choices, and you put yourself in charge. That's a good feeling—avoiding manipulation, being free of all the hype and half-truths, and using your brain to make sound, healthy decisions about your own body.

Does that mean you have to drive out into the country in search of organically grown vegetables and live on steamed cauliflower seven times a week?

Of course not. One of the benchmarks of a healthy diet is its *variety.* It *is* trickier than shouting "two cheeseburgers" into a drive-through speaker. You can't eat today's typical American diet and be fit, but you don't have to eat sawdust, either. Try to think in terms of whole foods—ones that *you* have to clean, cut up, spice and cook.

Can I eat my way to fitness, or do I have to exercise?

Nobody can be fit without regular exercise. Obviously. But it's no accident that the exercise section of this book falls between the nutritional and mental discipline sections. The physical work of building muscles and/or cardiovascular endurance is just one part of the package. All three elements are necessary. All three rely on each other. So I hate to single out any one of the three. If I had to, it would be nutrition. If someone is unwise enough to condemn himself or herself to the life of a couch potato—or if disability leaves them no choice—good nutrition will still improve health and fitness. And, to get back to the question: *Good nutrition will lead you toward exercise more than exercise will lead you toward good nutrition.*

That is a phenomenally important fact. Good nutrition is going to make you *look good* faster than exercise will. Not only will you decrease your bodyfat nutritionally, but you will need less sleep, your insulin level will be stabilized and your metabolism won't take you yo-yo-ing and roller-coastering through the day. Your body will feel better tuned and you'll have more energy for whatever you want to do—including exercise. It will also help you avoid the starvation-binge cycle that many people live on from day to day. Good nutrition alone is not enough, but it is a tremendous positive factor for fitness.

Mental discipline is something I'd like to say a few words about separately at the end of the book. But it's impossible to entirely separate mental discipline from nutrition. You cannot pick up new eating habits the way you pick up a suit from the cleaners. We are talking about a change of life. We are talking about a new personal understanding of reality, based on what food does to and for your body—not based on TV commercials, on what your friends eat, or on what the Hollywood stars eat. Nutrition takes an old truism—"You get what you pay for"—and stands it on its head. The fact is, you buy good nutrition with your brain and with your mental discipline, not with your wallet. You can eat well for pennies if you choose.

One restaurant I know in New York serves a well-marbled steak the size of a dump truck. The beef practically hangs over the table. It costs a *lot* of money. If the guy in the thousand-dollar suit with the steak knife in his hand is a good planner, he has drawn up a will. Because his idea of good nutrition is going to see to it that his heirs are spending the old man's money a lot sooner than he ever intended. Somebody at the next table, or at a little place down the street where the tab will be a whole lot smaller, is eating a tasty but healthy meal and enjoying it every bit as much. Why? Because they invested enough mental discipline to go against the flow and develop a new palate, one that's based on nutritional reality.

I see the mirror-opposite nutrition mistake that many women make—eating next to nothing. Their idea of a good diet is diet soda, lettuce, and bagels. America is full of such people starving themselves thin, when they could maintain a very nice bodyfat level with five times the volume of food—if they pick the right foods. Buck the trend—don't succumb to the emaciated examples in the media. The point is to be healthy and look healthy. There *is* a healthy way to look good and be lean. Besides, those rabbit-food diets are more often a setup for failure, leaving you tempted to give up the effort altogether. I recommend working on a healthier view of bodyfat.

Go *against the flow* is worth repeating. Because, in a nation with lousy eating habits, that is exactly what you must do. Going against the flow is never easy. Just look at the progress that has been made in cutting back on smoking. Now that it's cool not to smoke, there are converts all over the place. You can go *with* the flow and quit. As if we haven't known for years and years what a stupid and destructive habit tobacco is. When serious numbers of people look at a cheeseburger and an order of chili fries with the same disgust that they look at a cloud of cigarette smoke, then it'll be a whole lot easier to break the junk food habit. Society still doesn't make it easy to order an egg-white omelet with fruit instead of fried eggs with sausage and hash browns. There is nothing cool about getting your morning "nutrition" in a double-tall latte. Each time you sit down at the breakfast, lunch, or dinner table, you are going to have to work harder than you ever will in the gym. When you struggle to maintain that mental discipline, just go back the introduction to this book, face that mirror, and remember who you are doing this for. *You.*

These days, it's hard to imagine anybody being *totally* ignorant of the good nutrition message. Most everybody talks the talk, sort of. Fewer people are buying steaks the size of dump trucks. But often the message gets garbled into concoctions like diet soda and light beer, soy burgers topped with cheese and mayo, fat-free, nutritionally devoid pretzels, and grocery shelves full of other packaged products with "25 percent less fat and sodium!!!" (Still leaving you with 200 percent too much of both and *more* sugar than before.) The sad truth is that most of us remain functionally illiterate when it comes to nutrition.

For example, let's take the woman I saw in a Wendy's trying to do the right thing, nutritionally speaking. She pretty much symbolizes where we are in terms of what we put in our stomachs.

For starters, she was in a fast-food joint. That's no particular rap on Wendy's. They all present a challenge to anyone who wants to eat right. And did she ever try. She ordered the grilled chicken breast sandwich. Great choice. Lots of protein, low in fat. She ordered a whole-wheat bun. OK— slightly more nutrition than the white stuff. She ordered a baked potato, leaving behind the deep-fried french fries. Too bad the potato was the size of a Buick—starchy complex carbs are extremely dense. She only needed about one-fourth of that potato, and then she should have picked up the rest of her carbs from veggies. She was still on her way to her table as a winner, as far as fast food goes! But then she made that fatal stop at the condiment counter. What did she do? She poured ranch dressing all over her chicken and all over her potato. And not just a drizzling to add flavor—I'm talking a half a cup! Instant disaster. More calories, and more fat, than her chicken and bun and potato put together.

Of course, she could have chucked the whole thing and gotten a salad with grilled chicken and "light" Italian dressing. But then she would be consuming 1,200 milligrams of sodium, and the cottonseed oil in the recipe—while representing a low level of fat—would produce cholesterol in her body, helping to clog her arteries. Best alternative? Fix the same salad at home, with a homemade olive oil dressing.

It's a minefield out there, all right, with no quick fixes and no substitute for knowledge. A lot of nutrition consultants and weight-loss entrepreneurs would like to make it sound easy, almost like good nutrition is some kind of temporary inconvenience. They are preying on people's wish to just plunk down some cash and be fit and thin. Get out there and try that a few times, if you still want to believe it. But if you've been there and done that, then keep reading, because you know the quick fix never lasts.

Weight loss—meaning loss of bodyfat—is just one aspect of good nutrition. But it's a paramount concern for millions of Americans who spend billions of dollars in futile attempts to get weight off and keep it off. Chances are that bodyfat loss is one of your own concerns, one of the reasons you're reading this book. Chances are that you have tried not just one "diet," but many. Well, let me say up front that the word "diet"—as most people understand it—ought to be banned from the language. No temporary nutritional regimen can get you in shape, let alone keep you in shape.

Here is basically what I tell potential clients who come to me and ask me about nutritional counseling and personal training:

"It has taken you maybe 30 years to get the way you now look and feel. It will take a lot more than 30 days to turn it around. I'm not a magician. I'm not God. I can pass on to you the education and experience I've acquired. There's only one right way. I can give you the nuts and bolts. I can tell you how to do it. But until you get into the program mentally and emotionally, you are not going to see one physical change.

"After I talk with you and give you my written analysis, and you pay my fee, that analysis won't be worth the paper it's written on if *you* don't implement it. You have to *want* to be healthy—far more than you *want* those french fries or that cheesecake. That piece of paper gives you no sympathy, but it does give you 100 percent empathy. I've made my fee honestly and I'd like to see you lose weight, but only 30 percent of the people I've counseled follow through and do it. The successful ones get into the mental discipline part of it. They *want* fitness more than anything, and they focus on what they want. And they shape up and lose weight big time.

"I've watched many people transform in my gym—going from 300 pounds and red-line blood pressure to a 180-pound athlete that can run five miles. I've also seen very similar people given exactly the same set of tools make only 20 percent of that progress. I was teaching the same message, providing the same information, structuring an equally sustainable regimen for both. The difference? The successful ones had a deep *desire* to do it. They didn't just *want* to want it. And they wanted more than the attractiveness of a lean body—they wanted to be healthy. They had developed a deep, burning desire to take care of themselves. And they committed to it.

"I can provide information, experience, motivation—but I can't sit down with you at the dinner table and pull your hand away from the french fries, or go to the restaurant with you and order a grilled chicken salad or salmon with vegetables instead of the Coney dog with chili cheese fries.

"You need to make a commitment not with me, but with *yourself.*"

That's the unvarnished truth.

I do want to help you find the will to make a lifestyle change. Nutritionally speaking, I want to help you eat to live instead of living to eat. I want to provide some of the inspiration to get you into your own personal fitness program in whatever way works best for you. But you know what they say about 10 percent inspiration and 90 percent perspiration. You have to do your own perspiring. You have to eat your own meals. You have to make a commitment to yourself to be disciplined at the breakfast, lunch and dinner table. And believe me, that discipline, keeping that commitment, is far harder than *any* workout at the gym! I have seen people work like fiends at the gym only to erase all that work at the dinner table. You have to develop your own burning desire to be fit and keep your own inner fire lit.

That's one reason I used Part One to tell my story. Parts of it were not fun to tell. I like to think that a lot of readers will be smart enough if not inspired enough to say: "Hey, this guy's no genius. He had a debilitating disease. Damn near killed him. So he learned the hard way, by necessity. I think I'll get in tune with my body now, before it's too late."

If you are really ready to make that decision, you'll find that I'm about to give you the most basic, sane, realistic nutritional advice I know. No gourmet recipes, no emotional babysitting. Just the nuts and bolts. Because when you get a better grasp of *why* you should follow a healthy regimen, you're liable to be better motivated to get with it.

I learned all this stuff the hard way, for hard reasons. If you're lucky, your only reasons for learning it are to live longer, live better and fully enjoy your short little run on this planet.

That ought to be motivation enough.

9

What's in it for Me?

When you look at a well-prepared dish of food, what you see is something delicious like chicken Parmesan, shrimp scampi or linguini with clam sauce. Another way of looking at it would be to see dense, complex, "starchy" carbohydrates, plus protein, fat and cholesterol. The difference between those two visions is everything. I don't want you to lose the pleasure that comes with the first vision, and there's no reason you should. But if you want to be nutritionally fit, you'll have to start seeing the world of food through both lenses.

Looking through the analytical lens, I know exactly what goes into my body every day. I know by the gram, and in some cases by the milligram, what nutrients are stoking my fire. I am an extreme case, given my profession and my Crohn's. Even if you could tell me today that in no way would my physical appearance ever again have any bearing on my career, or that my Crohn's was cured and would never come back, I would still remain more aware of what I eat than 99 percent of the population. That's because I've learned from experience that the benefits reach far beyond developing a body that you can display on a stage.

I don't know how far you plan to go down the road toward personal nutrition awareness. Even if you're dead serious, you won't have to count grams of protein quite as closely as I do. You won't have to be as stopwatch precise as I am with my meals. You won't have to pass up quite as many "reward" treats as I do. But whether you are into a serious athletic regimen or barely exercising, you should have at least a working knowledge of basic nutrients. You should know what they do for and to you. You should know how to structure a healthy dietary regimen to fit your tastes and lifestyle.

So let's use this chapter to have a basic look, through that second lens, at all the stuff—good and bad—that you put in your stomach.

WATER

H_2O is the forgotten "nutrient." Many people are dehydrated and don't even know it. Not everyone who is tired, moody and fatigued is dehydrated, of course, but those are symptoms.

In one sense, water isn't a nutrient at all. Nutrients—the raw materials for fueling our bodies and building new cells—are found in food. But water is crucial to virtually every basic function of the body, from temperature regulation to blood circulation, metabolism, immune system function and waste elimination. The fact that something so basic can be so misunderstood or ignored shows just how far out of touch the average person is with his or her own body and its maintenance.

Take, for example, the matter of weight control—which always seems to be the one area where the average American picks up at least a passing interest in nutrition.

If you are overweight, or if you have fluid retention problems, you should be drinking *more* water. If you keep your body adequately supplied with water, it will actually speed up your metabolism. When the body is not being given enough water, it sees that as a threat to survival and—like a camel—begins to hang onto every drop. Drink more water, and the body will release the excess. Water also suppresses appetite, and naturally helps the body metabolize stored fat—so overweight people, with a larger metabolic load, need more water than thin people.

Every body, thin or fat, needs plenty of water every day. The average person loses about two cups daily through perspiration (temperature control), even without unusual physical exertion. Another two cups disappear in the respiratory process. The intestines and kidneys together use about six cups a day. That's about 10 cups total—not counting water loss through perspiration during any heavy exercise.

Some of that water loss is replaced through the food we eat, liquid or solid. The bottom line, however, is that the average person should be drinking at least six to eight cups of *water* each day. To be more specific, divide your bodyweight by two. That gives you the number of ounces of water you should be drinking. Divide that by eight to get the number of cups.

Be grateful to your kidneys, nature's filtering department. If you could somehow survive without them, you'd need to drink *2,500 gallons* of water every day just to flush out the system.

The fact is, millions of Americans don't come close to drinking their daily quota of water. Their rationale is that the oceans of pop, coffee, beer and liquor/soda combinations they knock down every day will do the trick. Well, there are some serious problems with that idea. Alcohol and caffeine, besides depleting the body of vitamins and minerals, are natural diuretics—meaning they actually lead to fluid elimination and dehydration.

There are many degrees of dehydration, of course. We're not talking about someone dying in the desert as his body runs dry. Lesser levels of dehydration occur when you don't take in enough water to replace all that's lost through breathing, urination and exercise. You don't have to be perspiring profusely or urinating frequently to be losing water. If you work in a stuffy house or office building, you lose large amounts of liquid invisibly. You can lose two pounds of water in the rapidly circulating cabin air of a three- or four-hour airplane flight. Stress, as well as alcohol and caffeine, acts as a diuretic. In other words, you can be dehydrating yourself on a *normal* day.

Speaking athletically—or in terms of any kind of physical performance—75 percent of muscle tissue is water. Dehydrate a muscle by 3 percent and you lose 10 percent of contractual strength and 8 percent of speed. Dehydration increases blood volume. Thicker, more concentrated blood stresses the heart. Your arteries become less able to provide muscles with nutrients and oxygen, and to eliminate accumulated wastes. So you don't need to be a scientist, rocket or otherwise, to figure out that dehydration is a common cause of poor athletic performance.

On the more cerebral side, dehydration can produce a minuscule but crucial shrinkage of the brain. Deprive yourself of enough water and your concentration and coordination will be affected.

In other words, you need those six to eight cups a day whether you're pumping iron in a gym or crunching numbers at a desk.

People often tell me: "No problem; I drink tons of water with my meals." Well, that is *exactly the wrong way* to consume your quota of water. It dilutes your food and makes for less efficient absorption of nutrients. If you drink milk, that is OK with meals because milk becomes a semi-solid in the stomach. But you should avoid water beginning 15 minutes before a meal; after a meal you should give your stomach 30 to 60 minutes to begin the digestive process.

Thirst, by the way, is a lousy barometer of whether or not you need water. Best to make water a habit. (You'll find that 90 percent of the battle with a dietary regimen is nothing but habit, so give it a chance.) Best of all, water is almost habit-*forming*. Just carry a bottle with you, and drink water throughout the day. For a few bucks, you can even pick up a squirt bottle with the volume marked right on it so you can easily track how much water you're actually getting.

Once you become water-conscious, you'll become fascinated by the stuff. In virtually any building in the United States you can turn a little handle and gallons of water come out—for pennies. Meanwhile, down at the supermarket, other kinds of water sell for several dollars a bottle. You need to know a little about both varieties.

Fluoride, for example, has been endorsed by the American Dental Association, and I haven't seen anything to convince me that fluoride in tap water will cause increased rates of disease. But, especially with children, I sometimes wonder if there isn't a fluoride overload in toothpaste, mouthwash and tap water. Chlorine, in sufficient dosage, is known to cause cancer. What's the bottom line with these chemicals in tap water? I wouldn't begin to judge whether you or I should avoid the water that comes out of any particular faucet. But I like to be aware of the fact that it's not a mountain stream pouring into my drinking glass.

Thousands of subdivisions and communities get their water from wells. Some wells produce hard water, some soft. In either case, it might have a peculiar taste. Chemically softened water is actually worse for drinking than straight tap water. Calcium and magnesium salts are replaced by sodium salts, adding as much as 100 milligrams of extra sodium per quart. Hard water, by contrast, contains relatively high amounts of distilled mineral salts that may help *prevent* heart disease.

In any case, even if your *source* of tap water is 100 percent pure and palatable, it might not be so pure by the time it gets to your kitchen faucet. Many Americans still are served by ancient underground pipes that add copper and lead to the water. And a single gallon of gasoline, if allowed to seep into the water supply, could contaminate the water of an entire small community.

What all this means is that home water purification may be something worth looking into. A $15 filter system over your tap isn't a bad bet. If you're serious about it, you could have a sample of your tap water tested. Or, more practically, you could do a little investigating to find out what kind of regular testing is done by your local officials. And maybe ask for a look at the results.

Bottled water is another story. Just because it costs a lot of money and portrays a pleasant rural scene on the label doesn't necessarily mean it's anything special. One survey showed that 93 brands of bottled water were being sold in New York. In most cases, the consumer couldn't really tell where the water came from or what was in it.

I always suggest that people launching a dietary regimen—a new eating lifestyle—start out drinking distilled water, at least for the first 90 days. Distilled water has many benefits, not the least of which being that it's relatively cheap. It helps flush out any unwanted mineral deposits from the body, especially if you've been drinking hard water for years. It is, literally, *pure* water; it functions almost like a detoxifying agent.

You could say that distilled water is "empty," but that's just fine. You ought to be getting your calcium and magnesium from green leafy vegetables anyway.

Drinking plenty of distilled water does exactly what those daily six to eight cups are supposed to do, no more and no less. It helps the body's organs go about their business. It's the lubricating oil of your personal engine. Your high-octane fuel—or low-octane junk—will come from the food you eat.

FAT

Fat has really gotten the yo-yo treatment in America regarding its relationship to health and obesity. Eating *some* fat in your food is essential to your health. There are extremists who will tell you that you can eat unlimited fat, as long as you consume no carbohydrates (we'll get into the potentially devastating effects of that approach later). There are other extremists who will tell you that *all* fat is bad, that it goes straight to your heart, butt and thighs. As with most things, the key is moderation and selectivity. Let me explain.

Scores of harmful and even fatal consequences have been solidly linked to high-fat diets—cancer, hypertension, cardiovascular disease and poor absorption of calcium from the small intestine, to name a few. Those risks are real whether you are obese or your constitution and exercise load have kept your body in pretty good shape. Keep in mind that most people on extremely high fat diets are also getting the wrong *kind* of fats—saturated fat and trans-fatty acids. It's harder to over-do it with the good stuff, like olive oil and canola oil. But it's easy to over-do it with the damaged fat of french fries, fried chicken, candy bars and movie-theater popcorn, or the excess saturated fat of fast food, cheeseburgers, bologna and bacon.

If weight loss is a concern, excess dietary fat is often the first culprit to eliminate. It's not like it goes directly to bodyfat; everything you eat has to be converted to glucose before your body can store it. But people typically find the worst stuff to be the tastiest, and consume it in mass quantities. Mass quantities mean mass storage if you don't use it. And besides the undesirable effects of weight gain, the "bad" fats will clog your arteries like a 100-year-old sink drain.

Fat-wise, the simple step toward using that second, analytical lens to look at food is to remember that there is visible fat and there is invisible fat. If you look at an untrimmed T-bone steak, you can see the fat as clearly as the spare tire on a couch potato. In our mostly shallow nutrition-consciousness, we're eating a lot less T-bone steak these days. But there is invisible fat in almost every corner of the menu, and we're not doing a very good job of avoiding it.

People who measure these things report that from 1910 to 1980, average per-capita daily fat consumption in the United States rose from 125 grams to 156 grams. What's even more interesting is that from the 1980's to 2000, we as a country significantly *reduced* our fat intake—many of us "got" the low-fat message and cut back. Yet Americans are more overweight than ever! So a diet that's "fat free" is not the magic key, and it is definitely not an excuse to load up on sugar and extra calories just because they're fat free. More on that later.

"Bad" fat is hidden in hundreds of foods, including most of America's most popular sandwiches and recipes. Margarine, butter, salad dressing, mayonnaise and altered oils account for 10 to 20 percent of the fat we eat. Red meat, poultry and fish account for 30 to 40 percent. Dairy products account for 15 to 25 percent. The rest comes from various sources such as nuts and eggs.

Almost everybody now is at least aware that there are three kinds of fat and two kinds of cholesterol, and that some are more user friendly than others. But most Americans don't retain much of that knowledge, and certainly don't act on it. They look only through that first lens and see the shrimp scampi instead of the fat and the cholesterol. The next few paragraphs include facts that *anybody* ought to know very well by now. Conversations I have every day with *health-conscious* clients convince me that isn't the case. So without going into great detail, we have to talk about what fat means nutritionally.

More than 90 percent of dietary fat arrives at the body in complex molecules consisting of three fatty acids: saturated, monounsaturated and polyunsaturated. Animal fats usually contain a high percentage of saturated fat. Keeping track of what kinds of fat you eat, however, is tricky. Beware, for example, snack foods whose labels proclaim "pure vegetable oil" as an ingredient. Coconut and palm oils contain even more saturated fatty acids than beef fat or lard. And don't be misled by "cholesterol-free" claims. Once digested, these oils do raise cholesterol levels in the blood. As you'll see, the simple—and effective—route is to limit your intake of fat of any kind. The fact is, that white stuff that borders your T-bone steak is fat, but so is the oil in your salad dressing.

Cholesterol is a wax-like substance that, in one form, clings to the walls of your arteries and makes them function like a water pipe gone bad. This can lead to heart attacks and strokes. Some studies suggest strongly that lowering levels of serum cholesterol also reduces the risk of cancer. Cholesterol is comprised of two groups of lipoprotein compounds—"high density" and "low density." HDLs have come to be known as the "good" cholesterol, because they actually draw the substance away from coronary arteries. LDLs are generally regarded as the predominant villain in heart disease. When your doctor tells you your cholesterol ratio, he or she is telling you what percentage of your cholesterol level is made up of HDLs. It's something worth checking.

A high intake of fat from red meats, eggs, dairy products and tropical oils—predominantly saturated—risks increased LDL (bad) cholesterol in the blood. It also increases the need for essential fatty acids, which can create a cycle leading to excessive bodyfat and other health problems.

Essential fatty acids are, indeed, essential in small amounts. Without them, the body cannot properly process and use the fats you ingest. Polyunsaturated fats—found in grains, seeds, nuts, soy foods and some vegetables—provide sequences of fatty acids called the Omega 6's and the Omega 3's. Your body's cells use these fatty acids to form membranes and conduct nerve impulses. Fatty acids are involved in hormonal function, brain function, aerobic metabolism and sexual wellness. Infants and young children need to consume somewhat more fat than adults. So getting the proper fat in the proper amount is crucial. But with such a wide variety of foods on our tables, rarely does anyone need to worry about adding vegetable oils to his diet.

In truth, nutritional science is still uncovering the nuts and bolts of fat and how it works in our bodies. For example, we know that the molecules of unsaturated oils—when hydrogenated for use in cakes, cookies, chips and other snacks—are rearranged into an unnatural framework that may cause health problems, even though they remain unsaturated. Margarine is produced from polyunsaturated fat, and is a cholesterol-free substitute for butter. But its chemical makeup may cause it to be associated with other health problems. On the positive side, recent studies suggest that olive oil and flax oil can reduce high blood pressure, stimulate pancreas secretion and lower levels of the (bad) LDL without lowering the (good) HDL.

So what's the answer?

Rule No. 1: Try to get at least two-thirds of your fat in the form of monounsaturated fats, from sources such as the following:
- Olive oil
- Canola oil
- Peanut oil
- Nuts (almonds, macadamias, cashews, peanuts)

The other one-third can be polyunsaturated fats. Saturated fats? Don't "try" to get your fat there. You'll get more than you need from lean meats.

Rule No. 2: Avoid damaged fats. If it is deep-fried or comes pre-packaged like in a candy bar, wrapped cake or muffin, or over a counter, it is probably damaged goods as far as your health is concerned.

Rule No. 3: Practice moderation. You need between 20 and 30 percent of your calories from fat each day—the healthy fats.

It's time to start reading labels, to buy a cookbook or two that lists fat content, and even to put a food scale on your kitchen counter. Start educating yourself—using the analytical lens to view food. Surf the Internet, and check out the Web sites of the fast food giants. You'll find the nutritional content of every single menu item. I warn you now: You are going to get some "sticker" shock—even from some of the supposedly healthy foods! Self-education on the subject of nutrition, you'll find, will not only improve your health, but it will be intellectually rewarding. Believe it or not, it will also be fun.

And *you* will be in control.

CARBOHYDRATES

Carbs might be the most debated nutrient of all. Again, there is an extremist on every corner, one telling you "no carbs," the other telling you "nothing but carbs." As with fats, there are good choices and poor choices for carbohydrates in your diet. A lot of research in the last decade has changed the picture of the body's reaction to carbohydrates. This research is also making the government rethink the food pyramid—that's serious stuff. First let's discuss some of the definitions.

All carbohydrates, simple or complex, are actually made up of one or more simple sugars. The most prevalent are glucose, fructose and galactose. Any one of these three alone is a monosaccharide. Join two together and you have a disaccharide. Glucose plus fructose equals sucrose, or table sugar. Glucose plus galactose equals lactose—the milk sugar that my own body rebels against so violently. Everything you eat has to be broken down to glucose before it ends up in your bloodstream, no matter what it was when you put it in your mouth—fat, carbs or protein.

Carbs, simple and complex, contain lots of glucose, the component that supplies many of your body's cellular needs. Glucose also helps maintain body temperature, regulate respiration, repair tissue and sustain the immune system. It is a critical part of your diet and I do *not* recommend any diet that eliminates carbs as part of some misguided weight-loss technique.

Let's look at how carbs are broken down and then either used as fuel or stored by your body.

To make a very complex process brief, your stomach breaks carbs down and releases them as glucose into your blood. The glucose is then either stored temporarily in the liver and pancreas or taken to long-term storage—fat. How does this "storage" happen? When your body "sees" the glucose entering the blood, it releases insulin into your blood. Insulin meets up with the glucose, picks it up, then takes it to the temporary storage area so it can be easily used for the next couple days. Sort of your body's own taxi service for energy. The insulin will carry *as much as you can store* to that "short term" parking lot (liver and pancreas), and you can use it for the next 48 hours. If you overeat, your liver and pancreas put out the "Parking Lot Is Full" sign, so the glucose has to go somewhere else. Our bodies, being the wonders of survival that they are, waste no energy. Whatever glucose is left over in your blood is converted and escorted as fat to your fat stores by the insulin. There is no rule-bending to be had—when the liver is full, it's full—even if it is your birthday or Saturday night or whatever other special occasion makes you overindulge.

The short-term parking really never expands significantly; it holds only just so much temporary storage. But your long-term parking lot—fat—can expand without limit. If you keep overeating, you'll just keep on expanding to store new fat. Very nice.

So how much fat you store from carbs is *partly* about the sheer quantity you consume. The other piece of that puzzle is what *type* of carbs you consume; certain foods trigger a lot more insulin to be released, and those are called "high glycemic" carbs. Having lots of insulin dumped into your blood is like having a lot more taxis ready to take the excess glucose to the fat depot. The more excess insulin you have in your blood, the better you are at storing fat. That's another strike against those starchy carbs and sugars.

So what about the *types* of carbs? We've all heard of "complex" and "simple" carbohydrates. *Complex* carbohydrates are carbohydrates with lots of long chains of sugars strung or wrapped together. Think bread, bagels, pasta, potatoes, vegetables and rice. *Simple* carbohydrates are made up of mostly the simple molecules themselves—stuff like fruits, juice, pop and candy.

Simple carbohydrates contain a lot of easily available glucose and other sugars. The process to break simple sugars down into glucose for your blood is simple compared to complex carbs—so they can get into your bloodstream fast, depending on how much fiber they have. Fiber is like a control meter. It slows down how fast the glucose can be pulled out of the food, because your stomach has to tear through the fiber first. Fibrous simple carbs are always a better choice than the refined ones—they enter your system at a more even rate. Plus, it's just plain harder to overeat fibrous carbs—just think how much easier it is to suck down a bag of jellybeans than it is to munch an apple!

Many simple carbs pack this double whammy—it's easy to eat them fast, and they turn to glucose fast. Things like candy, pop and juice are sugars with little fiber. One trip to the candy machine, and wham! Your blood is loaded. Another ride on the sugar roller coaster.

On the other hand, most fruits pack a fair amount of fiber. So although they are simple carbs, they take longer to eat and longer to break down than sweets. They are harder to over-consume than candy or pop. They do have a good amount of glucose, but the dump into your bloodstream is metered and controlled by their fiber content. The quick-reference tip is to pick a fresh fruit instead of candy, pop or juice when you crave something sweet.

Complex carbohydrates can basically be split into two more very important groups: starchy (dense) carbs and fibrous carbs. This is where advances from research of the last decade come in.

Starches and sugary foods have a chemical similarity. Starchy complex carbohydrates are, in a way, literally the sweetest of the bunch. That's because they are polysaccharides—a combination of more than two simple sugars. Some polysaccharides contain more than 1,000 glucose molecules linked together.

The "starchy" complex carbs include foods such as cereals, breads, rice, pasta, muffins, bagels and potatoes. These starches *do* provide the essential fuel—glucose, or blood sugar—for energy in every cell of your body. But why do starchy carbs get special attention? Because they are ultra-dense; it is easy to consume mass quantities of calories and grams of carbohydrates in a small package, like a bagel or bowl of pasta. You can exceed your caloric needs in minutes!

Starchy carbs are also typically low in fiber or refined, making it much easier to eat a large quantity quickly—think bagels versus broccoli. Then, without fiber to slow it down, the multiple glucose chains are easily and rapidly "unwrapped" in the stomach, and wham! Your bloodstream gets a dump-truck load of glucose. The typical American serving of pasta is almost double what the body can store short-term. So the insulin taxis come out in hordes, and you very efficiently store up the excess as fat.

Consuming large amounts of simple sugars and starchy carbs creates health and performance problems. Many are devoid of vitamins, minerals and fiber, and offer no nutritional fringe benefits whatever. Refined white sugar—sucrose—in the form of candy and pop head the American list of empty calories. It's followed closely by breads, pasta and rice. The simple molecules in sucrose require very little digestion and quickly take blood sugar levels above normal. Every office-working candy fiend knows the roller-coaster effect very well. It occurs when the pancreas secretes insulin to remove excess glucose from the blood, causing a *downswing* in blood sugar.

A high intake of refined sugars has been linked to elevated cholesterol levels, chromium deficiency, heart disease, diabetes and a laundry list of other problems. Alternatives such as fructose, maple syrup, honey or even juice concentrate are no bargain, either. Any energy from carbs that is not burned up immediately by your metabolism will be converted to fat. The simple fact is that excessive use of any sweetener is unhealthy.

So the point is once again, you have to bring out that other lens when you sit down at the breakfast, lunch and dinner table. This time, think in terms of equivalent glucose content.

Portion size is a major factor, too. Many people fall prey to the idea that if it's fat-free, it's a license for a feeding frenzy. Wrong! The average American dinner serving of pasta yields 800 calories. Your body can only use about 300 calories' worth of carbs in 90 minutes, and that includes your temporary storage banks! If you eat that bowl of pasta, you just cut a deal to wear the excess 500 calories on your hips, butt, thighs and gut. On the other hand, instead of the dish of pasta, you could have had a huge salad of fibrous carbs like broccoli, peppers, asparagus, string beans, tomatoes, cauliflower, romaine lettuce and spinach—enough to fill half a dinner table—and equal about 300 calories. Get the picture?

The average person needs about 45 to 55 percent of their calories to come from carbs—and not all in one sitting. Break those rules, and you've just signed up to wear the excess.

The bottom line is, get your carbs from unrefined, whole foods—colorful vegetables, fresh fruit, oatmeal, rye bread and maybe some occasional brown rice. The refined and dense stuff—even if it's fat-free—will rapidly fill your entire need for carbs, yet leave you unsatisfied and tempted to overeat. Pass up the breadbasket at dinner and grab a salad; pass on the rice and potatoes and ask for extra helpings of vegetables. There is such a wonderful, enormous variety of vegetables, you will never get bored! Got a sweet tooth? Downsize that cheesecake by splitting it with a couple of friends, and then try some high-fiber fruit. The key to enjoying your favorite "reward foods" is portion size!

The good news—and one of the most basic keys to planning what you put in your stomach—is that the stored energy from *complex* carbohydrates is available for *48 hours* before it is converted to fat. Is this an efficient energy source, or what? But remember, that only applies to what you can put into short-term storage. Once you exceed your body's limit, the insulin takes it straight to fat storage. After the digestive system turns carbs into glucose (or blood sugar), any of this energy that goes to the muscle cells must be metabolized and stored as muscle glycogen. A muscle cell can store about 90 minutes' worth of glycogen. Simple arithmetic shows you the value of up to 48 hours' worth of stored energy from complex carbs. It's a little more complicated than that, of course, and we'll talk about it later when we get into exercise.

PROTEIN

You might think that exercise builds muscle. Not exactly. Exercise actually *tears down* muscle tissue. Protein builds it back, bigger and stronger. You have to destroy muscle in order to build it. And you can't do that without protein.

Obviously, athletes and construction workers need more protein than office workers.

I just said a page or two ago that carbohydrates might be the most misunderstood nutrient. On the other hand, that honor might belong to protein. Generations of kids have had tons of red meat and peanut butter put down in front of them with the warning: "Here, you need your protein."

Yes, you do. But the odds are that you need less protein than you think, and that you're eating your protein *at the wrong time*. Protein is the building block to muscle, but your body is very finicky about how much protein it will accept at once.

During digestion, protein is broken down into amino acids. Twenty-two amino acids are known to be vital, and nine are known to be essential— meaning the body cannot manufacture them from other amino acids. That means they must come from your diet. And, since protein cannot be stored in the body like complex carbohydrates, you need a new supply each day. Furthermore, you need protein *several times each day*—including at breakfast.

Your body can utilize 35 to 40 grams of protein in a 2½-hour period. That's about 1½ chicken breasts. Any additional protein consumed within that 2½-hour period *will be converted to fat*. Yes, you can get fat by eating protein. No matter how nutritious the meal is, no matter how well you trimmed a cut of beef or chicken, no matter that you broiled it instead of drowning it in fat. Protein is a wonderful, necessary nutrient; but you must ration it to your body or you'll just be adding blubber.

Besides that, any excess protein that your body does not convert to glucose for storage must be eliminated as toxic waste. Athletically, this reduces performance and endurance. Athlete or not, a protein overdose will make you tired, increase blood acidity, dehydrate you and cause mineral loss—especially calcium. Meanwhile, excess protein consumption places a burden on your liver and kidneys.

In case you're wondering, yes, all those old training tables where an athlete "gets his protein" by chomping into one of those Godzilla-sized steaks are strictly from the Stone Age. After 30 or 40 grams, he is getting zero protein and consuming 100 percent fat or waste.

The protein secret for an athlete, or anyone who does strenuous exercise or labor, is to forget the whole idea of three square meals a day. You have to give your body protein in doses that it can handle. When I was in training for a competition, I'd eat *six* carefully planned meals a day. I'll explain all that later in detail. You needn't be that stringent or precise unless you're into competitive bodybuilding or high-performance athletics. The basic principle applies to everyone, however: Eating too much protein at once is worse than useless to your body.

There are many sources of protein. Red meat, in fact, supplies plenty of protein. But like most traditional sources of protein in the American diet, red meat also supplies too much saturated fat. The same goes for all that peanut butter mom encouraged you to eat, and to the yolks of all those eggs Americans chow down every morning. (Egg whites are another story; I eat them by the dozen.) Chicken breast is a good low-fat alternative. So is fish.

The body doesn't discriminate against vegetable protein, but putting a meal together is a lot trickier. Individual grains, legumes and vegetables lack adequate amounts of one or more essential amino acids. So the protein they supply is called "incomplete" protein. Vegetarians long ago learned to combine two or more foods to make a "complementary" protein, one that the body can utilize just as well as a steak or an egg—but without the fat. Beans and corn, for example, combine to make a complementary protein. Many Asian dishes combine vegetables with a moderate (by American standards) amount of beef, poultry or fish.

As you launch a healthy new nutritional regimen, one of your first steps will be to round up a few cookbooks that will show you hundreds of tasty ways to put together complementary proteins. You'll find that the basic recipe is to combine legumes (soybeans, lentils, kidney beans, blackeyed peas, chick peas, navy beans, pinto beans, split peas, lima beans and others) with grains such as barley, buckwheat, brown rice, oats or rye. It's delicious. And it's inexpensive.

Nutritional science has confirmed what some entire cultures have known for thousands of years: The need for huge amounts of protein is a myth. But we do need adequate amounts. I'll show you later how to calculate exactly the amount of protein you need to add to your diet as your physical activity rises. Athletes—and anyone who is building muscle by tearing it down—do need more protein.

VITAMINS AND MINERALS

I have my own vitamin company, but I'm not writing this to sell you my vitamins. Vitamins obviously are important to me, and so is this book. So let me say up front that Peter Nielsen is not the only person in the world with an ethical, well-planned line of vitamin supplements for sale.

The fact is, in a perfect world it would seldom be necessary to buy vitamin supplements—unless your doctor discovered a hereditary or illness-related deficiency. If you had lots of time to shop for produce and to prepare all your meals, or if you had a live-in cook, you could be reasonably assured that your diet would touch all the vitamin bases. The realities of modern lifestyles make it tough for many people to fit that description.

Today, the overwhelming majority of the food consumed in America is at least treated with preservatives for shelf life. Worse yet, much of our food is processed and packaged. We live in a fast-food frenzy, with nutrients cooked out of our food. We consume huge quantities of fat and sugar calories that are empty to begin with. In that environment, you would do well to educate yourself about vitamins. A good place to start is with the myths and misconceptions, which are many.

Vitamins are not wonder drugs. They are not food; you can't live on vitamins alone. That may sound like an obvious and unnecessary statement, but you might be surprised at the level of misunderstanding that exists. Many people, for example, think they can replace at least part of their food with vitamins. The fact is, the body cannot even assimilate vitamins without food. Pumping vitamin supplements into an empty stomach is the nutritional—and financial—equivalent of dumping them down the garbage disposal.

Vitamins contain no caloric value, no energy. They are no substitute for carbohydrates or protein or fat or water, or even for each other. You cannot become Mr. USA, or obtain the body of a fashion model, by skipping meals and popping vitamins. Not only do they supply no energy, they are not even a component of body structure.

Vitamins are not pep pills. They are substances that make the body operate in its peak *normal* fashion, not to hype it up and bring out unnatural performance. Just like protein, too much can be a bad thing—a very bad thing. An oversupply of B1, for example, can affect the thyroid gland and insulin production. Excess D can create an excess of calcium in the bloodstream. Megadoses of vitamin C wash out B12.

Simply put, vitamins are organic substances necessary for growth, vitality and general well being. Vitamins regulate metabolism through the enzyme system. They are crucial to your chemical balance, and a single deficiency can impair your entire body. Anybody who has been eating sugar, white flour, canned or preserved food, restaurant food that has been reheated, or fast food that has been sitting under a heat lamp has *some* level of deficiency. Most refined breads and cereals are high in nothing but carbohydrates. Enriched? Enriched with what? White flour is produced by removing 22 natural ingredients and, generally, replacing them with three B vitamins, vitamin D, calcium and iron salts. What comes back at you is hardly the staff of life.

Your lifestyle, and even your address, can rob your body of some of the vitamins and minerals (more on them in a minute) that you do get from your diet. Smoking cigarettes depletes vitamin C. Synthetic vitamin D in milk can deplete magnesium. Smog cover in a city leaves its residents with less vitamin D than rural dwellers get from the sun. Alcohol depletes B vitamins. Oral contraceptives can decrease the body's ability to make use of several vitamins. If you are eating a high-protein diet, you need more B6. That's just a sample.

Obviously, the idea of taking vitamin supplements isn't something to reject out of hand. Vitamins are one of the six important nutrients (along with water, carbohydrates, protein, fats and minerals). A simple working definition of all six is: absorbable components of food necessary for good health. Vitamins and minerals, because of their unique (some would say mysterious) role in that absorption, are a good place to get in a few words about the process. A quick refresher course on digestion will help you get that second lens in focus.

Digestion is a chemical process more intricate than any high-tech video game or computer program out there. It's about food, but it's not about award-winning cuisine. It's about nutrients. Your body begins chemically processing your food the moment you put it into your mouth, where an enzyme in the saliva called ptyalin begins to split starches into simple sugars. It's a 12- to 14-hour process for food to move through the stomach and intestines.

Virtually all absorption of nutrients occurs in the small intestine. That much you may remember from junior-high biology. What you may not remember, and may not have cared much about until now as an adult who wants to better understand his or her own nutrition, is the role played by a few other amazing organs.

The liver is a four-pound chemical factory. Once you're aware of its role and complexity, you'll think twice about punishing it with large doses of alcohol. The liver can modify almost any chemical structure sent its way, and it is a powerful detoxifying machine. It's also a blood reservoir and a storehouse for certain vitamins, digested carbohydrates and insulin, which is released to regulate blood sugar. Your liver manufactures your enzymes, cholesterols and vitamin A from beta-carotene. It plays a key role in the digestion of protein. And it produces bile, which contains salts that start the digestion of fats.

The gall bladder holds bile, modifies its chemicals and concentrates it tenfold. Just the sight of food can be enough to empty the gall bladder.

The pancreas provides your body's most important enzyme, insulin, which is injected into the bloodstream where it accelerates the burning of glucose and stores fat. The pancreas also secretes enzymes into the digestive tract to help break down fats, starches and protein.

You start to get the picture of how complex and wondrous this whole body engine is. I'm not trying to write a biology text here, but it's important to get some of these biological basics into your mind—and *keep* them there. Start thinking of food as the fuel for this engine and you'll be less susceptible to food impulses—to forgetting about looking through that second lens when you're contemplating a burger with cheese or a donut or that second or third beer. Vitamins are an intricate part of the enzyme system I just described. So are minerals, another minuscule piece of our nutrient intake but without which vitamins cannot function or be absorbed. The body can synthesize a few vitamins, but it cannot synthesize any minerals—the most important of which are calcium, iodine, iron, magnesium, zinc and phosphorous. About 18 minerals are known to be required for body function and maintenance, but many of them remain a mystery. Recommended daily allowances have been established for only six of them.

So where do vitamin supplements come from, and why are they sold in so many forms?

Most vitamins are extracted from natural sources. Vitamin A, for example, is taken from fish liver oil. B complex comes from yeast or liver. Vitamin E is usually extracted from soybeans, wheat germ or corn.

Tablets are the most common because they are easier to store and have a longer shelf life than powders or liquids. Capsules usually are used for supplementing oil-soluble vitamins such as A, D or E. Powders are used for extra potency. Many vitamin C powders contain as much as 4,000 milligrams in a teaspoon. And, for people with allergies, powders have no fillers or binders. Liquids can easily be mixed in beverages for people who have trouble swallowing pills.

Synthetic vitamins might be less likely to upset your budget, but in some individual cases, might upset your stomach. Both have produced satisfactory results, but in most cases I recommend natural over synthetic. Synthetic vitamin C, for example, is pure ascorbic acid. Vitamin C from rose hips contains the entire natural complex.

Chelation is also very important. It means the process in which mineral substances are changed into their digestible form. Huge percentages of many non-chelated products will pass through your body without ever being absorbed.

If you use vitamin and mineral supplements, store them in a cool place in a dark container away from direct sunlight. A few kernels of rice at the bottom of a bottle will work as a natural absorbent and guard against moisture.

Vitamins are organic substances and should be consumed with food and minerals for best absorption. The body works on a 24-hour cycle. Your cells don't sleep when you do, nor can they function without continuous oxygen and nutrients. For best results with vitamin and mineral supplements, space them throughout the day and take them after meals. If that's not practical, take half after breakfast and half after dinner. If you must take them all at once, do it after your largest meal.

The range of body functions that can be affected by a vitamin or mineral deficiency is enormous. Be sure to put them high on your list of topics for self-education.

AND A FEW OTHER THINGS

That's a thumbnail look at the six basic nutrients. But there are five other things that should be mentioned here. One of them is good, and Americans don't get enough of it. Four of them are bad, and Americans consume them by the truckload. First the good.

FIBER: This material, which comes from the cell walls of plants, plays a major role in digestion. It also plays a role in preventing heart disease and colon cancer. Like almost anything involved in publicized nutritional studies, food producers have jumped on the bandwagon with advertising and labeling. While that's OK, just make sure that any product touted as high in fiber isn't also high in sugar or sodium or fat. The best way to get your fiber is, as always, the natural way. Vegetables are chock full of it. Try steaming them to preserve the fibrous structure, instead of boiling them to death—which reduces the fiber benefit and often leaches much vitamin content.

As many as half of all Americans are afflicted with constipation or some form of gastrointestinal distress. Colon cancer is a leading cause of death. Meanwhile, underdeveloped nations whose people eat five to six times as much fiber rarely suffer from either disorder. Like many nutritional choices, the right one is simple and obvious.

Some fiber is water soluble, such as the cellulose in wheat bran and the pectin in apples, citrus fruits and certain vegetables. Other fiber—such as the hemicellulose found in whole grain and other vegetables—absorbs water. Both help promote a smooth and prompt passage through the digestive tract. And both help slow the absorption of glucose into the bloodstream.

A high fiber intake also helps shed excess bodyfat and may even lower blood pressure.

Eat a wide variety of fresh, whole foods and you'll get plenty of fiber in its various forms. The American Cancer Society recommends 25 to 30 grams a day; new research now recommends that you get even higher amounts—reaching close to 50 grams a day. But the average American intake is only 14 grams per day. Which tells you something about how much fresh, whole food we eat.

Now for the bad news:

SALT: After sugar, sodium chloride is the leading food additive in the United States. Excessive consumption has been linked to depression, bloating, weight gain, kidney disease and, of course, hypertension. The body needs about a quarter of a teaspoon per day. The American average is 20 times that.

Salt—like virtually all tastes—is an acquired one. Talk to people who, usually under doctor's orders, have drastically reduced their sodium intake. They come to *like* the flavor of whole, natural foods. Of course, they have to avoid the lines at the fast-food counter.

Our bodies can't function without the proper ration of sodium. But a regular diet contains plenty without adding a single grain of salt. Tomatoes and celery, for example, are high in sodium.

The recommended intake is 1,100 to 3,300 milligrams a day. One can of soup contains 900 milligrams, and the stuff is hidden in almost all processed food.

Sweating causes some sodium loss, but under normal conditions body reserves are not depleted—even in intense training.

CAFFEINE: This is one powerful legalized drug. Chances are you're not just enjoying your daily coffee and cola, you're addicted to it. Caffeine is intensely psychoactive. It acts directly upon the central nervous system and brings the body an almost immediate sense of clear thought, releases stored sugar from the liver and gives a feeling of relief from fatigue. That's the "lift" that comes with consuming the big three of caffeine: coffee, colas and chocolate.

The benefits are far outweighed by the risks. The release of stored sugar places heavy stress on the endocrine system. Heavy coffee users often become nervous and jittery. People shifting to decaf sometimes show withdrawal symptoms associated with drug users (and caffeine *is* a drug).

Some studies suggest that caffeine is linked to prostate problems and benign breast tumors, as well as to bladder cancer. It can rob the body of B complex vitamins, zinc, potassium and other minerals. It contributes to dehydration. It increases acidity in the gastrointestinal tract. Many doctors consider it a culprit in hypertension.

One article in the *AMA Journal* described a disease called "caffeinism," with symptoms including appetite loss, insomnia, chills, irritability and sometimes a low fever.

A lethal dose of caffeine is about 10 grams. How much are you getting, and where from? Here are a few sources, in milligrams: Coca-Cola, 64.7; Dr. Pepper, 60; instant coffee, 66; fresh ground, 146; black tea bags, 46; Anacin, 32 (relieve your headache and get a little boost); Dexetrim, 200 (maybe lose some weight; definitely get a little pep). That means three cans of Coke give you 2 percent of your lethal dose. If you dump in a couple of diet pills, you're up to 6 percent. Just keep that tally in mind as you order your afternoon double-tall latte.

Try some substitutes. Ginseng is caffeine-free and gives you a little lift. Herb teas can be invigorating. And water won't give you any caffeine, but you'll be doing your body a big favor.

ALCOHOL: In recent years we've become a lot more conscious of the carnage alcohol causes on our highways. Less publicly, alcohol abuse causes even more long-term carnage within our bodies. A good argument can be made that alcohol abuse is our greatest drug problem.

Alcohol is not a stimulant; it's a depressant. It does not warm you up; it increases perspiration and loss of body heat. It destroys brain cells by dehydrating them. It depletes the body of numerous vitamins and minerals. Four drinks a day are enough to cause organ damage, to hamper the liver's ability to process fat.

With today's new awareness, you don't need to be told how much bad news lurks in alcoholic beverages of any kind. But it's worth a reminder. Even in moderation, by the way, alcohol is a major negative to athletic performance.

EPHEDRA: This is possibly one of the most dangerous developments in the crusade for "quick fix" weight loss in our country. Several major brands of so-called diet pills contain ephedra, and some pack caffeine and other stimulants on top of that, all in the same pill. If you use this substance, you may be taking your life into your own hands.

The U.S. government is considering a ban on the product, based on a growing number of wrongful-death suits brought against manufacturers who use ephedra in their products. Several makers have pulled ephedra, or products containing it, from the market in light of these allegations.

If you are in the process of trying to retrieve, improve or maintain fitness, please don't veer down the "quick-fix" path, derailing your efforts to make real and sustainable changes in your health habits. You have come this far in taking responsibility for your health and lifestyle, don't chuck it all now by falling prey to the "just take this little pill" mentality.

At best, you're tossing away your progress and the mental discipline a healthy lifestyle requires; at worst, you could be playing Russian roulette with your life.

If you use it, you should know the risks. Consult with your doctor. A wealth of information is also available online (see the resource listing at the end of this book). Sure, products containing this substance work. Chances are that if you take it, you'll lose weight—but possibly a lot more.

IO

Not Weight Loss, But Fat Loss

I expect that some readers of this book are obese couch potatoes. I expect that others are hard-core weightlifters or marathon runners who, in addition to their exercise regimen, have adopted a realistic and healthy nutritional lifestyle. I suspect that most readers fall somewhere in between. That's a *big* range, and I'm going to offer some fitness tips for all of you. Meanwhile, if you're already flat-bellied and if your ideal weight is what you see whenever you step on the scales, then you might want to pass this chapter on to somebody close to you who has a weight problem.

You can't write any kind of fitness book in America without including a chapter on nutrition and weight loss. We are a *fat* country, despite all those slim bodies we see in TV commercials for everything from beer to soda pop to cheeseburgers. The food America eats pretty much guarantees that most of us will be overweight and/or artery-clogged even with a moderate amount of exercise. Take away the exercise and we'd be an *obese* country. The truth is, you can't find many Americans who don't "want to lose some weight."

The key word is "want." How badly do you "want" to lose weight? Maybe you "want" a luxury sedan, a condo on the beach, and a mansion on the hill with a Jacuzzi and an in-ground pool. Those things don't come easy because they cost about 100 years of the typical paycheck. A slim and fit body—which will give you more real pleasure and long-term benefit—doesn't cost a dime. It's there for the taking. So do you "want" it or not?

I've made a decent life out of turning negatives into positives. And there is no way, without the Crohn's and all that agony, that I would have found myself pumping iron and posing my body. One of the most consistent paradoxes in life is how we can be blessed by adversity.

Like I said earlier, the beautiful thing about life is that, as long as your mistakes aren't so big that they kill you, it gives you a chance to try again. And that's the way you have to look at an out-of-shape, run-down body. Specifically, in this chapter, a *fat* body. Don't look at it as a prison that you're stuck in; look at it as *a catalyst for change*. The worse shape you're in, the deeper your desire to change.

Most people who come to me for nutritional counseling and personal training are seriously overweight. They're not bad people, they're fat people. In fact, I've met some incredibly nice people, some lifelong friends, while doing PT. And the nature of the business pretty much guarantees that my clients are successful. People usually don't hire a personal trainer and nutritional consultant unless they're making a dollar or two. Such people are almost universally frustrated beyond belief that they can lead a sales staff to great success or manage a company, but cannot manage their own bodies. Considering that very few things in life are as important as the body that a person must live in, it does say something about the human condition, doesn't it?

People pay me for counseling and training and then miss sessions. I can't do anything about that. People come up with cockeyed rationales for why they're in the shape they're in—most often, "genetics." More baloney. They don't really *want* to lose weight, and I couldn't do it *for* them if I were their nutrition consultant *and* personal trainer for 10 years.

That's why I give each potential client the talk I outlined in Chapter Eight, the one where I explain it's all up to them. Then, before getting on to the nuts and bolts of nutrition and weight loss, I try to explode a number of myths:

MYTH No. 1: "My mother's fat, my father's fat, I'm fat. It's inherited. I was *born to be fat.*"

FACT: Yes, some people genetically inherit a tendency to form extra fat cells. If they want to be slim, they have to work a *little* harder at it. But not all basketball players are seven feet tall. And obesity is *not* inherited. Obesity is caused by eating too much of the wrong foods, skipping meals(!) and forgetting about exercise and stress management. Fat cells then load up with fat and you, as they say, "get fat." Fitness and nutrition will overcome genetics every time. That doesn't necessarily mean that you can look like a fashion model or an NFL wide receiver, but that's not what we're talking about.

MYTH No. 2: "I can't lose weight because I don't have the discipline to starve myself and ignore hunger."

FACT: This is probably the most tragic of all the myths, because if you are eating the proper foods there is no reason whatsoever to be hungry. You can be "full" and still lose weight. Hunger is your body's way of saying:

"Eat." Make yourself artificially hungry and you'll gorge yourself with artificial food. Sugar binges, carb binges, fad diets and crash diets will rob your body of water or muscle tissue and actually make it easier for your body to accumulate fat. Try fad diets long enough and you could run away and join the circus as Starvini, the Human Yo-Yo.

MYTH No. 3: "I'm in great shape except my hips, so I'm going to spot reduce."

FACT: You *can't* spot reduce. If you're happy with everything about your body except your waist, or hips, or thighs, or buttocks, then you have to lose fat, period. Your body and your metabolism are symmetrical, even if the mirror tells you otherwise. If you lose weight, you'll lose it throughout your body. Specific exercises can strengthen certain muscles, but that has nothing to do with bodyfat accumulated in the same area. The best overall exercise, by the way, is aerobic—burning excess fat throughout the body by burning calories.

MYTH No. 4: "I'm not going to think about nutrition to lose weight. I'm going to pick an aerobic exercise—swimming or cycling or running— and I'm going to do it every day. The food part will take care of itself."

FACT: Neither nutrition alone nor exercise alone is the way to lose weight. You have to pay attention to both. The fact is, if you lead an active life—and don't spend hours and hours sitting on the couch—nutrition alone will come closer to doing the job. If you train every day, your body will benefit, no question. But the fact remains that eating 3,500 calories adds a pound and burning 3,500 calories subtracts a pound—and the wrong kinds of calories can really accelerate that addition process. You could be an aerobics maniac, but if you sustain on junk food, burgers and starches, you will still become fat. And you cannot exercise away an overdose of cholesterol or pump iron to reverse the damage of alcohol abuse on your liver.

MYTH No. 5: "I'm not emotionally equipped to lose weight."

FACT: This is one of those hot-button issues. I respect the struggle of the many people who desperately want to shed fat but find themselves see-sawing between emotional stress and eating binges. It's a vicious cycle, and the emotional complexities of overeating are real. I'm not a psychologist, so it is beyond the scope of this book to address the causes of obesity and weight gain that result from emotional or eating disorders. Although much benefit can be gained by the approach of this book for an eating-disordered person, I leave those issues to professionals qualified in that area.

For the many other folks who frustrate themselves daily with failed attempts to eat properly, I do know that gaining fat itself becomes a source of stress, because they often feel like a failure. Stress sets them up for even more overeating. If you keep on with the same approach, eventually anyone would conclude that they just "don't have what it takes."

You have to climb out of that trap.

The idea that you "can't" lose weight due to lack of mental fortitude or will power *is a myth*. Will power, when it comes to overeating, is a macho concept akin to pouring all of your decision making into one crucial, vulnerable moment—when temptation is at its worst. If you don't make a plan and follow it, you'll take the path of least resistance every time—which usually means junky food. Your mom probably put it best: Never go grocery shopping when you're hungry. Apply that to your whole week. It's all about proper planning, commitment, and yes, self-discipline.

When I say commitment, I'm talking about taking the time to make decisions about nutrition *ahead of time*—not waiting till you're ready to wolf down an entire pizza by yourself. Self-discipline is about following through, every day—taking the time to shop for groceries, avoiding the pig-out restaurants, ordering the healthier dishes. It's just plain self-sabotage to rest all hope for your health on a split-second decision when you have all week to plan it right.

Like I said, I'm not a psychologist. But I know from repeated first-hand experience that learning how to make good choices nutritionally by understanding *why* they should be made produces results. And it's not just the waistline that improves. A lot of self-esteem comes along for the ride.

Now for some nuts and bolts. The first thing to do is to forget about time and forget about your bathroom scale.

You forget about time for three reasons. First, you didn't get fat overnight and you're not going to get thin overnight. Second, in this diet-crazy country, 90 percent of the weight-loss schemes you've ever seen or heard of—hundreds or even thousands of them—lie about that simple first fact. So-and-so's quick weight-loss diet. So-and-so's 14-day artichoke plan. Forget it. It's all nonsense. Third, the only time we're talking about is *the rest of your life*. We're not going to switch your car from kerosene to gasoline for a few weeks. This is a permanent switch to the fuel you should have been pumping in the first place.

Forget about your bathroom scale for just one reason. We're not really talking about weight loss (though you probably will lose weight if you have a serious weight problem). We're talking about *fat* loss. You want to lose weight fast? It's easy. Dehydrate yourself. That's what a lot of fad diets do. Most of your body is water, so shedding a few pounds quick is a snap. Stupid, but a snap. Or how about muscle? Muscle weighs more than fat, and it's easy to shed muscle. We can sit you on a couch, deprive you of protein and get rid of some serious pounds in a flash.

Since muscle weighs more than fat—and since you might be adding some muscle from the exercise side of your fitness equation—a moderately overweight person might actually *gain* weight while shedding fat. In any case, I think belt notches and dress sizes are a far more accurate measure of "weight loss" than any bathroom scale. After a month or two on a healthy nutritional regimen, you'll be seeing your progress in the mirror instead of looking at a couple of ticks on a scale that might mean nothing except that there's a little less water in your body today.

Next comes the old—and highly controversial—question: "How much should I weigh?" There's no absolute, easy answer. One study at Harvard Medical School suggests that being even moderately overweight is more harmful than generally believed. In fact, people weighing at least 10 percent below average for their frame showed the lowest death rates. Another study by the National Institutes for Health showed the same results—as long as the below-average weight was not a result of illness, of course.

If you want to seriously pursue this business of how much you "should" weigh, there are a lot of different approaches out there. You can spend a lot of money on an electronic bodyfat meter or pay a doctor or clinic to measure it the same way. You can get most health professionals to measure it using a caliper and a scale—for a modest fee.

If you're not scared off by arithmetic, you can estimate your own body mass index (BMI). It's not highly accurate, but it's free. Here's what you do to calculate your BMI:

1. Convert your weight into kilograms by dividing your weight (without clothes) in pounds by 2.2.

2. Convert your height in inches to meters by dividing your height (without shoes) by 39.4; then square that number (multiply it by itself).

3. Divide your weight in kilograms by the square of your height in meters. That number is an approximation of your body mass index.

As an example, take a man who is 5-foot-10 and weighs 200 pounds. Divide 200 by 2.2 to get 90.91 kilograms. Divide 70 inches by 39.4 to get 1.78 meters. Square 1.78 to get 3.168. Then divide 90.91 by 3.168 and you have a body mass index of 28.69.

Another example could be a woman who is 5-foot-6 and weighs 160 pounds. Her BMI would be 25.77.

For women with average musculature, a BMI above 23 often indicates overweight. For men, it's a reading above 24. Obesity (20 percent above the normal range) begins at 27.2 for men and 26.9 for women.

That's all pretty complicated and not very accurate. I still think that well-toned muscles, a strong heart and an ability to look in a mirror without flinching are the truly meaningful measures of a body's fitness.

Traditionally, the measurements that launch any weight-loss program are the weight-for-age-and-sex charts and the calorie charts. People check out the weight chart, then start counting calories and stepping anxiously on the scales. My own view is that if losing bodyfat were as simple as counting calories, then shedding blubber would be as easy as skipping breakfast. A lot of people do just that, and fail.

Three variables really determine what you are going to weigh:

1. Your energy balance—the number of calories you consume each day (input), compared with the number of calories you burn (output).

2. The type of calories you consume—for example, high versus low glycemic foods.

3. Your body composition—your percentage of bodyfat compared with lean tissue. That's because your energy output depends on your basal metabolism rate (BMR), the rate at which you burn calories while at rest. And *lean tissue is more active than fat tissue in burning calories.*

Obviously, exercise is a key part of this picture. Anaerobic exercise builds lean tissue. And aerobic exercise will raise your BMR for hours after you are through exercising—meaning you'll still be burning calories.

Nutritionally speaking, there is one critical fact about nutrition and BMR that blows away all of the myths about "dieting."

Spacing your caloric intake throughout the day—throwing away the "eat three square meals by the clock" tradition and eating five or six meals a day—will *raise your basal metabolism rate.* Your body's fat-burning activity will be elevated for almost all your waking hours. The hormonal signals that cause fat cells to multiply will be reduced. In other words, here's yet another reason to think less about how much you eat and more about *what* and *when* you eat.

Remember also that the body can utilize protein only in relatively small, rationed quantities. And that simple *and* starchy carbs are cheap, junky fuel good for a quick high and a quick crash—and for conversion to fat if consumed in excess. So what about all of the diets out there that tout a "magic ingredient"—like no carbs, or the beet-and-rutabaga diet? Where does that leave you in the search for your best dietary friend? Right. A proper balance of protein, fat, and carbohydrates. No magic answers. A zero fat diet won't do it. Neither will a zero-carb diet.

What you want is a diet consisting of about 45 to 55 percent low-glycemic carbs, plus 20-30 percent "good" fats, and the remainder of lean protein.

And don't eat it all in one sitting. You should spread each of these nutrient groups out—through the day—in three modest-sized meals plus two or three snacks.

My nutritional consulting clients almost invariably assure me that they eat a wide variety of food. Usually it turns out to be a wide variety of fat-drenched foods and an excess of empty or starchy carbohydrates. One way to replace the sense of food deprivation, real or imagined, is to take a real run at the enormous variety of fruits and vegetables that you probably don't try very often. To stimulate the taste buds, use new herbs and spices as replacements for the fats that you remove from your diet. To get your "good" carbs but still retain some of that "comfort food" feeling, try bean salads, green beans, lightly sautéed mushrooms, low-fat coleslaw and hummus, just to name a few examples.

High-quality nutrients in vegetables, legumes, whole grains, fruits, fish, poultry and non-fat dairy products make it easy to keep a lid on caloric intake without getting into calorie-counting mania. I strongly caution against any "diet" that aims to drastically reduce calories, such as the under-1,200 calorie diets that are popular in some circles. If you go that route, do it only under the guidance of a doctor. If you choose to limit yourself to 1,200 to 1,800 calories a day, make sure that you are getting a reasonably accurate count. The best guide is "Calories and Your Weight," available from the U.S. Government Printing Office. Calorie-counting software can also be purchased for your home or office computer.

A gram scale for your kitchen isn't a bad idea for keeping track of fat- or protein-dense foods such as meat and poultry. After a while you'll be able to eyeball a piece of meat fairly accurately. But at first, you won't believe your eyes. It doesn't take much meat to cross the line from protein consumption to fat production.

You'll also do well to sort out the difference between "hunger" and "appetite." Hunger is an unpleasant physical sensation caused by an urgent need for food. Appetite is a desire to eat whether or not you are hungry. Your appetite might need discipline, but you should never be hungry. Remember that appetite is affected by habits, social situations and emotional pressures. In the early stages of your new nutritional regimen, you might have to plan strategy just like someone who is shaking the nicotine habit—avoiding situations that trigger your addiction.

Make a production out of quality instead of quantity. Put on some music, get out the tablecloth and relearn how to have conversation while you're dining instead of just stuffing your mouth.

You've heard a million times that you should relax and eat more slowly. Why? Partly it's to give your digestive system a break, instead of forcing it to treat every meal like an emergency rush job. But another reason is that it will take less food to leave you feeling satisfied and "full." There are hormonal reasons for this. Suffice it to say that it takes about 20 minutes for the insulin in your cerebral spinal fluid to send a "full" message to the brain. You can eat a reasonable amount of food in 20 minutes and be full. Or you can eat like a demented hog for 20 minutes and be full. Your choice.

That little scenario is complicated for obese people, whose insulin generally enters the bloodstream more slowly—meaning it takes them longer to be satisfied. Take smaller bites. Pause longer between bites. Take *control.*

Empty the house of junk food. You're not going to be eating it any more and you won't be doing friends and loved ones any favors by feeding it to them. One good way to come up with new dishes and snack recipes that will keep *you* happy is to scour the cookbooks and your own imagination for recipes that will please *them.*

Drink lots of water between meals. And remember that even though you're probably going to be eating more often under your new regimen, an evening snack consisting of a little protein, a little carbohydrate and a touch of good fat will keep your metabolism going as you sleep. Four p.m. is the cutoff for your limited intake of starchy carbs and sugar—evening time is *not* the time for those treats.

Try keeping a diary of what you eat and drink. Memory won't cut it when you want to reconstruct a picture of a day's, or a week's, nutrition.

The bottom line is that we're talking about behavioral change and your *feelings* about food. Just as with your behavior and attitudes in any area, there is no substitute for education. You don't tend a garden, maintain a car or learn to play piano on impulse. You learn and practice. You care about what you are doing and pay close, regular attention to it. Where your body is concerned, you can never learn too many why's and how's. They will help you keep viewing a plate of food through that second, analytical lens. And don't let a setback or a lousy nutrition day ruin your outlook. We all have them. You can start your nutritional day over at any time of day and get right back on track.

Planning is key; if you have all the ingredients for a quick, healthy meal ready to pull out of the fridge and go on the stove or in the oven, you have just bought insurance against that deadly swing through the drive-thru.

If you just can't curb your appetite, ask yourself if you're dehydrated. Even mild dehydration is a major setup to overeat. People often mistake the brain's thirst signal for hunger and grab a candy bar or some chips. Which, by the way, still leaves you dehydrated.

Mood swings and stress are real enough. Try, for starters, to channel them somewhere besides your mouth. I assume you don't come home and kick the cat. That's good. Now start thinking about the fact that you shouldn't come home and eat a quart of ice cream, either.

This is one of several areas where exercise becomes a super partner to nutrition in weight loss. Instead of taking it out on that quart of ice cream, take it out in a long brisk walk, or a jog, or a tennis game, or a swim—or whatever exercise fits your taste and your current body condition.

Frustration, boredom, a loss of motivation—these kinds of emotional swings occur in all of us. We get stalled by mental blocks and psychological factors that I'm not qualified to analyze. But I do know that we have to prevent them from slopping over into what happens to our bodies. If you arrive at one of those negative plateaus, it is vital that you take immediate, constructive action.

Often I'll choose a new form of exercise or an increased level of activity. That'll boost my metabolism and help fight boredom. (If you're not a weightlifter, believe me, there are times when all those reps *do* get boring.) I also try to add something new to my diet. Any change of pace—expanding your social network, meeting a new friend, becoming more involved in a project or a hobby—can help get your goal-orientation back on track.

Rewards are important. Sometimes we forget how often we reward ourselves with food. So it'll help immensely if you consciously replace hot fudge sundaes and pizzas with non-edible rewards. Get out to a movie. Get out to the bookstore and buy a new book to read for pleasure. (Load up on nutrition books, but avoid any that include phrases like "14 Days," "Easy" or "Miracle.") Buy earrings. Go to a concert. Get a new CD and enjoy. *Bon appetit* doesn't always have to mean food.

I I

Fueling for Performance

Nutrition and exercise go hand in hand. What you put in your mouth directly affects what you can do with your body. Most of that picture is the long-range effect. Downing one can of spinach may have helped Popeye lift Bluto off his feet with one arm, but the benefits of good nutrition are not quite that immediate for the rest of us. The "one candy bar equals one winning drive to the basket" that you see in TV commercials is definitely a poor and misrepresented picture of the fuel-performance relationship. Physical performance is all about energy, but it's *not* about mainlining a blue sports drink to win the NBA playoffs.

Muscles use energy, which they ultimately derive from glucose. The more you use your muscles, the more energy they consume. Sustained exercise of your most important muscle—your heart—will use even more energy. That's why aerobic exercise—putting your heart and lungs into overdrive, fanning the calorie-burning flames with oxygen— will help you trim your body. Assuming, of course, that you're eating right.

Your body can get fuel for exercise from several sources. The most direct source is complex carbohydrates. The digestive system turns carbohydrates into glucose. When this blood sugar is transported to a muscle, it becomes glycogen and is stored there for energy—about 90 minutes' worth. Different kinds of exercise—at different levels of intensity and duration— determine how much energy you use, how quickly you use it, and whether you are burning muscle glycogen, blood glucose, or two secondary sources of energy.

One of these secondary sources (good news) is fat. Depending on the kind of exercise you are performing, exercise *can* burn up fat.

The other source (bad news) is protein. If your body is burning protein for fuel, that means two things: one, you are extremely fatigued, and two, your body is feeding on itself.

Anaerobic exercise is an intense thrust of energy for a matter of 10 to 15 seconds. Traditional weightlifting exercises are anaerobic. Those heavy, quick bursts with the weights build and strengthen muscle, but the anaerobic pathway allows muscles to utilize only one kind of energy: muscle glycogen.

Aerobic exercise elevates the heart rate and sustains it. Generally, it takes 15 or 20 minutes of exercise to get your cardiovascular system up to speed. Spinning, aerobics and kickboxing are just some of the types of classes offered at gyms. And participants are actually burning glucose 18 to 19 times faster than the powerlifter in the next room doing 10 quick presses with a 200-pound barbell. And, as you'll see in a moment, the aerobic exercisers can actually burn up fat—*as long as they don't get too intense in their workout!*

Cross-training, a combination of both aerobic and anaerobic exercise, builds strength *and* endurance. This is a golden pathway to fitness through exercise, and we'll talk about it extensively in Part Three.

Light to moderate exercise—up to 60 percent of cardiovascular capacity—can be fueled almost entirely through the aerobic pathway. Hormonal changes and decreased insulin output promote the release of fatty acids from fat tissue into the bloodstream. These fatty acids, combined with fat pools in muscle tissue, supply about half the energy for low to moderate exercise. Muscle glycogen and blood glucose supply the rest.

During high-intensity exercise—70 percent or more of aerobic capacity—the body does not use fat as fuel. Fat simply can't supply energy fast enough for high intensity exercise, with the body straining to supply enough oxygen to match its workload. Glucose delivers about five calories per liter of oxygen and fat delivers only 4.65 calories, so the body shifts to glucose and glycogen as an energy source. The accumulation of lactic acid is another reason for the shift. Lactic acid, a waste product of high-intensity exercise, hinders mobilization of fatty acids from adipose (fat) tissue.

Duration of exercise also plays a major role in whether or not you burn up any fat in the gym or on the road. Muscle glycogen is the predominant fuel for the first 30 to 60 minutes of most types of exercise. It takes that long for fatty acids to be freed for use as fuel. The longer you exercise, the greater the contribution of fat tissue to your energy consumption. If you exercise moderately for four to six hours, fat can contribute as much as 70 percent of the calories you burn. The longer you exercise, the less intense it must be.

The basic nutritional message is that if burning up fat is one reason you're about to step on a treadmill, you're not interested in blocking or delaying your body's switch to fat as a fuel. *The pre-workout dose of complex carb energy is not the proper strategy for weight loss.*

Ironically, the more fit you are, the easier it is for your body to burn fat. Nobody ever said life was fair. There's scientific proof of this. Endurance training increases an athlete's ability to perform more aerobically during exactly the same exercise—in other words, to use more fat and less glycogen. When I said the body starts to accumulate lactic acid at about 70 percent of aerobic capacity, I was referring to people well along in a fitness regimen—individuals in training. For an untrained, out-of-shape person, lactic acid starts to accumulate at about 50 percent of aerobic capacity.

This point at which the lactic acid starts building up is called the anaerobic threshold. Increase your anaerobic threshold and you'll increase your ability to burn up fat instead of glycogen. Obviously, your athletic performance in any kind of sustained event will also improve greatly. And there's a double bonus. Trained (fit) individuals also can store about 1½ times as much glycogen in their muscle tissue. So they have more glycogen to begin with, and will burn it up at a slower rate.

Even the leanest marathoner stores more bodyfat than he or she will ever need during exercise. If you're dieting, you have probably figured out by now that your new nutritional lifestyle means you will be burning a lot of glycogen. Right. Your goal is to increase the use of fat as fuel through endurance training, not by eating fat.

CARBOHYDRATES AND PERFORMANCE

Stores of muscle glycogen begin to reach low levels in high intensity exercise that exceeds 90 minutes. When glycogen reaches a critically low supply, the body leaves the athlete two choices: slow the pace dramatically or collapse from exhaustion.

Glycogen can also be depleted in a slow process over several days of repeated heavy training, when you do not eat enough carbohydrates to replace what you've used. When this happens, glycogen stores drop each day—and the athlete wonders why he's not able to maintain his training intensity. That's often the explanation for a "stale" feeling in an exercise program. Instead of the "overtraining" that often gets blamed, it's an insufficiency of carb intake—and sometimes dehydration. That doesn't mean you should eat three baked potatoes at a sitting; it means that your consistent intake of the proper amounts of non-starchy carbs (as well as protein and fat) is critical to performance. Training increases the amount of all nutrition you need, but it is not an excuse to wolf down huge plates of pasta on a daily basis.

(To be specific, if you're in advanced training, we're comparing a 40 percent carbohydrate diet with a 70 percent carbohydrate diet during repeated days of two-hour workouts.)

In one study, fit athletes who started out like gangbusters on an intensive training program were not able to perform even level exercise after seven days on a low-carb diet—with muscle glycogen stores dropping each day.

"Training glycogen depletion," to use the textbook phrase, happens to athletes involved in exercise other than endurance training in the gym. Football, basketball and soccer players—any athlete who uses repeated near-maximum bursts of effort—can experience the same type of exhaustion. Telltale signs are inability to maintain normal exercise intensity and a sudden weight loss of several pounds. Lack of carbohydrate intake and lack of rest days are culprits.

If you are in serious training, you should be eating a diet rich in fibrous complex carbohydrates and you should be taking periodic rest days, during which your muscles will replenish their stores of glycogen. I preach this so much that you'd think the Complex Carb Sales Board was paying me off. But our newest nutritional failing is an onslaught of diet "experts" pushing a "no carb" diet—to counteract our excess intake of empty and starchy carbs. Not only are both approaches dangerous to your health, both leave you unable to exercise properly.

And one more word about simple vs. complex carbs. Yes, simple carbs also provide glycogen synthesis. But fibrous, unprocessed, complex carbs provide more nutrition—including fiber, iron and B complex vitamins necessary for metabolism. Most importantly, the "good" complex carbs are time-released and will not turn to fat if not burned up immediately. My own recommendation is a non-training diet of 45 to 55 percent carbohydrates—of which 10 percent can be simple carbs from fruits and juices and 10 percent from starches.

CARBOHYDRATE OVERLOADING

Carb overloading is not always a negative phrase. It refers to an athletic strategy for nearly doubling muscle glycogen storage before an event. The theory goes that the greater the pre-exercise glycogen content of the muscle, the greater the endurance potential. Even if you're not a competitive athlete, you'll probably find the nuts and bolts of the strategy interesting.

There's are two ways to do it.

The old way—which I tried for a time myself—was basically an exhaustive weeklong training regimen, followed by a precise exercise and nutrition regimen for the last six days before an event. For the first three days of the last six, the athlete would consume a *low*-carbohydrate diet while continuing to work out, thus lowering muscle glycogen storage even further. Then, the last three days before the event, the athlete would rest and consume a *high*-complex carbohydrate diet to promote muscle glycogen storage and super compensation for the depleted stores. During those last three days, the athlete would consume about 100 calories of complex carbs per hour.

For many years, this was considered the optimal way to achieve maximum glycogen storage. But it had some serious drawbacks. For one thing, you could develop hypoglycemia (low blood sugar) while starving yourself of carbs. You could also develop ketosis (increased blood acids), with side effects like nausea, fatigue, dizziness, diarrhea and irritability. Live and learn. Like I said, I was my own guinea pig from the day I came out of the hospital. Many of the things I've learned came the hard way.

The newer and improved version of carb loading makes more sense, and it provides muscle glycogen stores equal to the old, disproved method.

Six days before competition the athlete exercises strenuously—to 70 or 75 percent of aerobic capacity—for 90 minutes. On that day, and for the next two days, he or she consumes a normal diet of 40 to 55 percent carbohydrates. On the second and third day, the training is decreased to 40 minutes. For the next two days the athlete eats a high complex carbohydrate diet (about 70 percent) and reduces training to 20 minutes at 70 percent of aerobic capacity. On the last day, the athlete rests while maintaining a high complex carbohydrate diet.

This modified loading method allows you to maintain high intensity training longer, but will not affect pace for the first hour of your event. Runners who used the loading method for one 30K event doubled their glycogen levels. Both groups "ran their race" for the first hour, but the carbohydrate-loaded group was able to stay on a faster pace longer in the latter stages of the race.

The old-time carb loading method used a carb starvation period because it was thought necessary to trigger maximum levels of glycogen storage. Now we know better. *Endurance training* is the primary stimulus for muscle glycogen production and storage. The exercise to deplete storage, by the way, must be the same exercise as the event that you are preparing for. That's because glycogen is depleted—and manufactured and stored—in the muscles you use. So a runner, for example, needs to deplete storage by running, rather than by cycling.

In the final three days, when the athlete tapers training activity, he needs a high complex carbohydrate diet because these are the real "loading" days of the regimen. That's why it's essential to reduce training during this period. Otherwise, he or she will use too much of the stored glycogen and defeat the whole scheme.

For those that have difficulty downing all that oatmeal, vegetables, fruit and such, commercial carbohydrate supplements are available. But beware—diabetes or high triglycerides combined with carb loading can lead to medical complications. Athletes with these conditions must check with their doctor before trying the regimen.

Each gram of glycogen a person stores also means water storage. Some athletes report feelings of stiffness or heaviness as a result. In bodybuilding, that's just fine—because muscle is 75 percent water. The more glycogen you store, the more your muscles will fill with fluid and the more they're going to look "ripped" or "cut"—well-defined. Remember, you won't have this water between skin and muscle; you'll have it *in* your muscle.

CARB INTAKE BEFORE EXERCISING

While you are exercising or performing athletically, the body relies on pre-existing glycogen or fat storage for energy. A pre-exercise meal or snack won't do anything for you immediately, but the carbohydrates can add to blood glucose—and energy—if you exercise for more than an hour. That's why athletes who compete in a prolonged endurance event that relies heavily on blood sugar won't perform as well if they skip breakfast. The overnight fast lowers their liver glycogen storage, the main source of blood sugar.

In the past, athletes have been discouraged from eating on the morning before training or a competition. Common advice is to eat two to three hours before exercising, so if there's a morning track meet or an early appointment at the gym, most people will skip breakfast. The rationale is that any food remaining in the stomach at the start of exercise might nauseate you when blood is diverted from the gastrointestinal tract to the exercising muscle. Athletes also have been advised to avoid high-carbohydrate meals immediately before training on the grounds that higher insulin levels might cause hypoglycemia or fatigue. Actually, there is a great range of personal reaction here. Some athletes in endurance training are insensitive to lowered blood sugars (I'm one of them). There's really no substitute for experimenting with your own body's reaction to pre-exercise meals.

The simple fact is that eating before exercise can help restore depleted liver and muscle glycogen storage. If gastric emptying is a concern, then you can always try a commercial liquid meal. They're high in carbohydrate calories, contribute to hydration and can be consumed nearer to the time of a competition because of the shorter gastric emptying time. They may help *prevent* pre-event nausea in a tense athlete. Liquid meals also are more convenient during daylong competitions, such as track meets, triathlons or tennis tournaments. Just remember to include your proper balance of protein and fat as well.

How much carbohydrate should an athlete eat before an event? The consensus suggests one to four grams per kilogram of bodyweight, consumed one to four hours before exercising. To prevent possible gastro distress, decrease the intake if you eat nearer to the time of the event—four grams per kilo of bodyweight four hours prior to the event, down to one gram one hour prior to the event.

Good examples of pre-exercise carbohydrate foods: oatmeal, fruits, juices and non-fat yogurt.

What about consuming simple sugar before exercise? Studies on the subject are all over the map. For sure, consuming a candy bar before anaerobic exercise—such as weight training—will not increase performance because your body already has plenty of glycogen stored for the activity. It could be useful, however, for a long-distance runner who will need energy when muscle glycogen falls to a low level. Again, there are great individual differences here. You should test your own reaction in training.

FLUID INTAKE BEFORE EXERCISE

For peak performance, you should be fully hydrated before training or competing. Drink 16 to 20 ounces of water through the two hours before training, and drink another 16 ounces of cold fluid 10 to 15 minutes before starting.

Drinking the full quota of fluids just before exercise can produce hyper-hydration. Some people think hyperhydrating improves thermoregulation by shortening the usual delay in sweating and decreasing the quantity of sweat. No serious advantages have been proven for this strategy, however. Particularly in hot weather, I'd suggest an athlete should drink no more fluid—probably about 20 ounces—than he or she will be comfortable with.

What kind of fluid? More than 15 minutes before exercising, stick with water. In the final 15 minutes, water-diluted fruit juice or a sports drink is a good choice if the activity will be longer than an hour.

I shouldn't have to tell you that caffeine is a lousy pre-exercise beverage.

FLUID INTAKE DURING EXERCISE

Individual responses vary tremendously. Drinking fluids during exercise is as much an art as a science, even though there are tons of reports on the subject. In any case, fluid replacement during exercise—training or competition—is vital to prevent thermal damage. In training, it helps you get into a routine for drinking fluids during competition.

You should aim to replace at least 50 percent of fluid loss while you exercise. Drink four to six ounces of fluid every 10 to 15 minutes. Cold fluid (40 to 50 degrees Fahrenheit) will help cool the core body temperature and will leave the stomach more rapidly than warm fluid. Warmer fluids make sense if you're exercising in cool or cold weather.

The idea is to replace lost fluids, so one of the prime attributes in choosing a drink is that you find it palatable. If you like it, you'll drink it. Water is palatable to most anyone. Water also is inexpensive and easily absorbed. Good stuff, that water.

Sports drinks combine glucose and sodium to promote rapid absorption from the small intestine. That's OK. Just remember that any benefits of carb replacement are strictly limited to endurance activities. If you drink juice, it should be diluted at least by half.

CARBOHYDRATES AFTER EXERCISE

You know that eating adequate amounts of carbohydrate during intensive training is vital to replenish muscle glycogen stores. The time period when you eat after exercise is also important. The sooner the better.

The only serious study I've found on the subject measured muscle glycogen production when two grams of carbohydrates per kilogram of bodyweight were consumed immediately after exercise, two hours after exercise and four hours after exercise. Two hours after exercise, glycogen production was cut by a third. Four hours after exercise it was cut by 45 percent.

There are several possible explanations. Blood flow to the muscle is greater immediately after exercise. Muscle cell is more receptive to glycogen. And the cells are more sensitive to insulin, which promotes glycogen production.

Commercial complex carb drinks can make sense here, because many athletes are not hungry for a meal after heavy exercise.

How much should you consume after heavy exercise? The best evidence suggests about 400 calories (or 100 grams) of carbs within 15 minutes of a workout, but you still have to get your protein and a little fat somewhere.

FLUID INTAKE AFTER EXERCISE

Intensive exercise blunts the sensation of thirst, and it will be quenched before you replace the fluids you have lost in a workout or competition. That's why you're got to be deliberate about fluid replacement after your event or workout. For every pound of bodyweight lost, you should drink about 16 ounces of liquid. Start drinking as soon as the workout is over—even before you shower—then keep drinking at a comfortable pace.

The temperature of what you drink is less important at this point, but a warm drink can prevent hypothermia on a cold day of outdoor activity.

If you undertake moderate exercise in moderate temperature, you're going to lose more water than electrolytes—meaning water is the crucial nutrient to replace. Plain water is fine. A sweet-tasting fluid has only the side benefit of stimulating you to drink more. Alcohol or caffeine—in coffee or soda pop—are diuretics, and will only make you lose more water.

Fluid replacement generally follows the same principles no matter what your activity, but some sports need special consideration. Fluid should never be restricted for football players, for example. In hot weather, exercising underneath all that gear can generate incredible fluid loss. Endurance runners and cyclists must drink fluid while running or pedaling. Protecting against dehydration is such an important factor that runners and cyclists must learn to function with fluid in their stomachs, even if it's a personal discomfort. Swimmers—who bury themselves in water—lose pounds of the stuff while sitting around in the sunshine between events.

In some quarters, two particular sports raise fluid deprivation to a near-criminal level. Boxing and wrestling are based on weight classifications, and the easiest way to make weight is to shed water. It's dangerous and stupid.

Water plays a key role in athletic performance by maintaining blood volume, which is necessary for cardiovascular function and for regulating body temperature. Thirst is an unreliable barometer of your hydration. That's why athletes—and recreational competitors—should follow the guidelines above.

Fluid replacement is even more important with the very young and the very old.

Children have lower heat tolerance, a lower sweating capacity and a lower cardiac output—which makes it harder to dissipate excess body heat. In cold temperatures, their extremities are more likely to freeze. Kids should drink 10 to 14 ounces of fluid before going out to play. I know it sounds impractical, but a boy or girl playing in warm temperatures should continue to replace fluids at the rate of about three ounces every 10 to 15 minutes during activity.

As for older people, one survey found that after 24 hours of fluid deprivation, 67- to 75-year-old men were less thirsty and drank less water than 20- to 31-year-old men. Besides which, many older people are taking many medications—often including diuretics. Fluid consumption needs to be carefully monitored as we grow older.

12

The Building Block to Muscle

Protein is the royalty of nutrients. It is found in some of our highest-priced foods. (It's also found in some of our lowest-priced foods, but they tend to get snubbed—as if you couldn't possibly find a *protein* living at that address.) Many people eat unhealthy meals every day, confident they are doing themselves a favor because they are loading up on protein. It is, after all, the stuff that builds muscle.

Several generations were raised on nutritional folklore that went something like: "Protein is real food; the rest of it is junk and fattening."

The fact is, protein *is* the royalty of nutrients. But to have a healthy relationship with protein you must treat it like royalty. Protein has a very limited schedule, and you must accommodate it. If you are building muscle, through weightlifting or otherwise, you absolutely must take a scientific approach to protein consumption. Otherwise, you will be tearing yourself apart when you think you are building yourself up.

Anaerobic exercise *breaks down* muscle tissue. Your musculature then replaces itself with larger, stronger tissue—if you are consuming the proper amount of protein *at the right time*. Since the body can utilize just 35 to 40 grams of protein in any 2½ hour period, sitting down and gorging yourself on protein will produce nothing but fat and toxic wastes. So the amount of protein you consume through the day must be carefully adjusted to fit your exercise regimen. The more muscle you tear down, the more protein you need to replace it. The less you exercise, the more you need a common-sense diet of complex carbohydrates.

This protein connection also often explains why crash diets fail—or even boomerang—leaving the puzzled dieter weighing more than he or she did in the first place. A tremendous lowering of caloric intake for an extended period lowers the basal metabolism rate (BMR), making it difficult if not impossible to continue shedding body fat. If you foolishly go on a starvation diet while exercising, and deprive yourself of protein, you will *lose muscle* instead of fat. I can guarantee you that losing muscle will not produce a great loss in size—just a lowering of your metabolism and tone.

While in training, it is absolutely essential that you eat *four, five or even six meals* a day—not just for the other nutritional benefits of that regimen that we have talked about, but to get protein to your muscles. If you eat more than 40 grams of protein in any 2½ hour period, you might as well be pouring the precious stuff out on your driveway.

So what's an accurate, practical way of selecting and monitoring your protein intake? How much protein is enough?

You'll read advice ranging from one-half gram of protein to a full gram of protein per pound of body weight—a 100 percent variance!

The chart at the end of this chapter—multiplying your ideal body weight by your activity load—tells what's right for you.

I use exactly the same formula. Because I'm a bodybuilder in training and do a tremendous amount of intense anaerobic exercise, I need a large amount of protein. The way I get it is by eating six carefully planned meals a day, none of which look like anything out of a Norman Rockwell Thanksgiving scene. (You'll see a daily menu example in the next chapter.) This is the *only* way I can get the protein I need. It *must* be spaced through the day.

If you're a weightlifter, or training intensively in another sport, you can follow my program out the window and benefit greatly. If you exercise moderately, lightly, or not at all, this will strike you as one bizarre-looking regimen. But remember, my goal here is not to get every reader eating chicken breasts three or four times a day. It's for you to understand how the body accepts protein, and how you must incorporate that into your own nutrition regimen—whatever your physical workload.

How to Determine
Daily Protein Requirement

GRAMS OF PROTEIN PER DAY, DEPENDING ON ACTIVITY LEVEL
(Multiply by ideal body weight, using chart below.)

.5 grams per lb.: Sedentary, no sports or fitness training
.6 grams per lb: Jogger or in light fitness training
.7 grams per lb: Sports participant or moderate training three days a week

.8 grams per lb: Moderate training every day, aerobic or weights
.9 grams per lb: Heavy weight training daily
1.0 grams per lb: Heavy weight training daily plus sports training, or
two-a-day weight training

Ideal Body Weight	Total Daily Protein Grams					
	.5	.6	.7	.8	.9	1.0
90	45	54	63	72	81	90
100	50	60	70	80	90	100
110	55	66	77	88	99	110
120	60	72	84	96	108	120
130	65	78	91	104	117	130
140	70	84	98	112	126	140
150	75	90	105	120	135	150
160	80	96	112	128	144	160
170	85	102	119	136	153	170
180	90	108	126	144	162	180
190	95	114	133	152	171	190
200	100	120	140	160	180	200
210	105	126	147	168	189	210
220	110	132	154	176	198	220
230	115	130	161	184	207	230
240	120	144	168	192	216	240

So here's how a pro bodybuilder—me—uses the same protein guidelines that you can adapt from the chart:

Let's say 190 is my ideal body weight. If I were not involved in sports whatsoever—didn't even jog—I would need protein by a factor of .5 grams times 190, or 95 grams of protein a day. If I were into jogging—or light fitness, training maybe once a week—I would need .6 grams of protein times 190 (114 grams of protein a day). Training three times a week, I would need .7 grams (133 grams total). Training daily with weights or aerobics on a moderate basis, I would need .8 grams (152 grams total). And if I were into heavy weight training every day, I would need .9 grams (171 total). In the last 12 weeks before a competition, doing a double split of exercises, I would need one full gram per pound of ideal body weight—or 190 grams of protein a day.

At 27 grams per average boneless, skinless chicken breast, and three grams per one large egg white, and 30 grams per typical broiled unbreaded fish filet, we're talking about a lot of chow. You might literally get tired of eating. In that case, to reach your quotas, you'll probably want to supplement your food with egg white powder or commercial amino acid powders. (As always, you shouldn't drink water from 15 minutes before a meal until 30 to 60 minutes afterward, or you'll have absorption problems.)

I carry a log with me and keep close track of those protein grams, and the times that I consume them.

If your protein intake matches your needs and your fat intake is low, you are doing exactly what is needed on the nutritional side to acquire tremendous muscle definition. The muscles you break down anaerobically come back bigger and stronger with the aid of your careful protein intake.

In the fall of 1991, I saw a tremendous difference in my own body from the Southeastern USA competition to the Mr. World competition. My body fat was 4 or 5 percent for the USA on October 5, and on November 23 it was 2.5 percent for the Mr. World. What I did was increase my protein intake from .75 gram to one full gram per pound of ideal body weight. At the Mr. World I had more size, more "cut" and had less fat on my body.

Don't forget: This didn't happen because I guzzled protein. It happened because my protein intake matched my very heavy training load, and was spaced so that my body could use it.

13

So What's on the Menu?

I'm not in the cookbook business or the diet business. I wouldn't want to try to come up with a year's worth of recipes and peddle it as "Peter Nielsen's 365 Days to a New You." That would be a waste of time. For one thing, only one reader in 100 would follow the regimen to its conclusion. That's why this book concentrates on *motivation*—on trying to show you so many good reasons for taking care of your body that you won't need a prescriptive cookbook under your arm in the kitchen and a personal trainer looking over your shoulder to make you exercise. For another thing, there's so much variety out there that a one-size-fits-all prescriptive diet won't work. Too much variety in people, too much variety in food.

Among people, there is first of all variety in taste. I grant you that if you are in the depths of a fat-laden, starch-heavy eating rut, you'll need to acquire some new tastes and modify some behavior. But you can eat healthy and still have plenty of elbow room for staking out your own preferences.

People also have enormous variety in exercise load. Now that you've seen some of what that means nutritionally, you know it wouldn't make sense to prescribe you a "diet" even if every reader was a 29-year-old male, 5 foot 10 and 180 pounds. If the heaviest weight you carry is a briefcase, and the farthest you run is to catch the Good Humor truck, then you need to look at a different menu than someone who is in a gym for an hour every day.

A third great difference among people is dietary abnormalities. That doesn't affect most people. But because of my lactose intolerance—and because of the nutritional counseling I do—I'm aware that the number of people with special problems is far greater than generally recognized. If you're lucky, it can be a blessing in some ways. I wouldn't have a pizza or an ice cream problem even without will power; any dairy product makes me sick.

The variety in food—when you get into real food—is awesome. I mean, the difference between T-bone, New York strip and pot roast doesn't add up to much when you compare it to the zillion ways you can dress up shrimp or chicken. Red meat is red meat and fat is fat. I can cook chicken breasts more ways than there are bars in Brooklyn. If you want, I can make them look like ravioli. Fresh vegetables come in and out of season, keeping you creative and keeping you from being bored. Once you realize what non-fat dairy products are all about, you'll be able to slop white stuff all over your steamed veggies without guilt.

So it really would be pointless and counter-productive to do the cookbook thing here. But after all this fact and philosophy about nutrition as it relates to exercise, it might be useful to give you a couple of examples of healthy menus for two very different kinds of people. For good measure, I'll throw in a day's example of my own training diet.

A major key to success with any new nutritional regimen will be to put a little effort and creativity into tapping all that variety. There's an infinite number of ways to come up with menus that will offer the same nutrition. Remember what all these menus have in common is getting the saturated fat out, getting the starchy carbs down and the fibrous carbs up, and fitting—and timing—protein consumption to match activity load. Those attributes are far more important than calorie-counting.

Goal-setting is a wonderful thing. And consciously thinking about what you put in your stomach should be one of your goals for the rest of your life.

THE COUCH POTATO FAMILY PLAN

Here's four days' worth of a new eating regimen for your typical out-of-shape American who hasn't given much conscious thought, and no action, to a nutrition and fitness regimen. If you are overweight, you could actually use these menus exactly as written. More important, you can analyze the principles behind them and draw up your own.

Calories for each day add up to the 1,900 range. Unless you have a real obesity problem, I don't recommend any regimen that drops calorie intake to much less than 10 times your weight.

Chances are these menus show a drastic reduction in fat and carb calories compared with what you're eating now. That's probably the single most important part of this plan. Veggies and fruits are high. Protein is from low-fat sources.

Remember to drink plenty of water through the day, but don't use it to wash down your food. In a perfect world, you'd bypass water with meals. If you're absolutely hung up on it, bring a small glass to the table and *sip*.

These menus deliberately plan for you to eat five times a day. Planning multiple mini-meals will help control your appetite, will see to it that when you eat, you are eating good food, and will keep your metabolic rate higher. Be sure to never skip breakfast, and then to space each meal throughout the day.

Remember, if you are a serious couch potato with typical American eating habits, you will feel better and lose weight on this type of nutritional regimen—even if you don't launch a formal exercise program. Without exercise, however, you will *not* become fit. The beauty is that if you eat this kind of food every day, your body will start leading you toward exercise. Nothing radical about that. Somebody with a 50-pound spare tire isn't real likely to hop off the couch and suggest a brisk walk down to the park and back.

DAY ONE:
BREAKFAST
¾ cup (cooked) of oatmeal (not instant)
1 cup low-fat milk
(if lactose intolerant, skip milk and increase egg whites to 6)
4 large egg whites
½ banana
Hot beverage

There's nothing like breakfast cereal to tune up your label-reading ability. What you don't want are sugar and sodium. Lots of cereals that tout high "enrichment" are loaded with both. Plain old-fashioned oatmeal is a great choice, as is barley. Most of the rest of what's out there is sugar and empty processed carbs. The simple act of reading "breakfast food" ingredients can go a long way toward raising your nutritional consciousness.

"Hot beverage" is, of course, a euphemism for coffee. I've already preached my sermon on caffeine. If you're hooked, try to withdraw gradually. Cut back consumption. Give ginseng or herb tea a chance.

The cup of low-fat milk can be split between your cereal and your hot drink. If you've been drinking whole milk for 30 years, low fat is going to taste empty. What you're missing is *fat*. Dairy fat is fat, just as sure as the stuff in your frying pan. After a few weeks, you won't be able to stand the taste of whole milk. It'll taste like, well, *fat*.

SECOND BREAKFAST (2-3 hours later)
½ apple
¼ cup low fat cottage cheese *or* 1 ounce turkey

LUNCH (2-3 hours later)
½ cup tuna, packed in water
1 tablespoon low-fat mayonnaise
2 slices rye bread *or* large veggie salad plus 1 piece fruit
Lettuce, onion

Even today, store shelves are about equally filled with oil-packed and water-packed tuna. The latter gives you virtually fat-free calories of protein. The former takes the same thing and pours on the fat. More label reading. More consciousness.

Maybe you don't like onion. Maybe you do like tomato. Maybe you like dandelion greens! Whatever garnish you like from fibrous fresh produce, pile it on.

Rye bread is really the only minimally processed bread. Lots of factory-produced bread dodges the issue. "Wheat bread," for example. Of course it's wheat bread; we assume it's not made from zucchini. But is it whole grain? Seek out the real thing and after a week or two you won't be able to stand the puffy, fluffy, empty white stuff. Your digestive system will thank you.

AFTERNOON SNACK (2-3 hours later)
Small peach
1 ounce low-fat cheese *or* soy hotdog

See, this is the way diets read. "Small peach." Is it a *big* deal whether it's "small" or not? No. The big deal is that it's a peach, and not a chocolate bar or even a granola bar. Is it a big deal that it's a peach? No. Don't buy a bushel of peaches. Buy a few peaches and a few apples and a few kiwis and a few grapes—whatever. Variety is not only the spice of life, it's a cornerstone of good nutrition.

DINNER (2-3 hours later)
4 ounces chicken breast stir-fried with two teaspoons olive oil and ½ cup or more of mixed veggies—bell peppers, broccoli, snow peas, mushrooms, onions, carrot slices.
¼ cup brown rice
Large salad with one tablespoon olive oil or flaxseed oil dressing

Baked apple

If you're not already into stir-fry, you'll get there quickly. For one thing, it's delicious. For another, it's one of the easiest ways to be creative.

Scour the cookbooks for seasoning suggestions, then invent your own. Use a Teflon wok, or other synthetic-surfaced utensil, to get by with the least amount of oil.

Olive, peanut and canola oils for cooking are a great way to get your healthy fats. Remember, good fat is essential to health. And an easy mixture of balsamic vinegar with some olive oil is a great dressing.

EVENING SNACK (2-3 hours later)
Small fruit
¼ cup low-fat cottage cheese *or* 1 ounce turkey sausage

DAY TWO:
BREAKFAST
Egg-white (6) omelet
½ cup fruit
½ cup (cooked) oatmeal (not instant)
6 almonds

You've got to be serious to get into separating eggs and tossing the yolks. But that is the one and only way to get out the cholesterol *and* fat. The frozen egg substitutes are indeed better than whole eggs if you can't handle it. But you know what? I've been eating egg whites only since I was a teenager and they're delicious. Funny how food works that way. Habit. Habit. Habit.

To be specific, here's the difference between a whole large egg and the egg white alone. Fat: six grams in the whole egg, 0 in the white. Cholesterol: 274 milligrams in whole egg, 0 in the white.

SECOND BREAKFAST (2-3 hours later)
8 ounces low-fat milk *or* soymilk

LUNCH (2-3 hours later)
8 ounces low-fat yogurt *or* 3 ounces chicken breast
1¼ cups strawberries
Salad with one tablespoon olive oil dressing
2 whole wheat bread sticks

SEMI-MEAL (2-3 hours later)
One-half of a whole wheat pita stuffed with chopped veggies and sprouts, 1 ounce of low-fat cheese, and garnished with spicy mustard

DINNER (2-3 hours later)
6 ounce flank steak
1 cup green beans
1 cup cauliflower
Seasoning to taste
1 small kiwi fruit

The butcher shop used to keep the flank steak in the back room. It wasn't the thing you'd display with the traditional fatty cuts. Flank steak has moved out of the closet in a more nutrition-conscious era. Learn to cook it, and it's a good pacifier for somebody who grew up on beef twice a day. A few ounces are plenty, for example, to make a stir-fry downright beefy. It is still beef, and it does contain saturated fat—though much less than other cuts. Limit your six-ounce steak to a once-a-week treat.

EVENING SNACK (2-3 hours later)
1 ounce low-fat cheese
¼ cup applesauce

DAY THREE:
BREAKFAST
1 grapefruit
½ banana
¾ cup low-fat cottage cheese *or* 3 ounces turkey
Hot beverage with skim milk

SECOND BREAKFAST (2-3 hours later)
6 ounces protein drink
½ cup applesauce
5-8 peanuts

LUNCH (2-3 hours later)
Bowl of vegetable soup
3- to 4- ounce grilled chicken breast
Small baked potato with ½ cup non-fat yogurt

If you get into cooking soups at home, you can control the fat and sodium content pretty easily—and make a delicious, storable meal while you're at it. If you eat soup from a can, buy the lowest-fat, lowest-sodium brand you can find. If you're in a restaurant, you're at the mercy of the chef. Obviously avoid creamy or cheesy soups. Don't be afraid to ask what's in the soup—or any other dish. There finally are enough health-conscious people around that any decent establishment knows by now it must be able to answer its customers' questions.

If you know you have a genuine low-fat or even nonfat bowl of vegetable soup in front of you, feel free to put a *light sprinkling* of grated parmesan on top.

Baked potatoes are a super-dense source of carbohydrate, so consider a small one to be a treat—and never after 4 p.m.

DINNER (2-3 hours later)
Seafood primavera with three ounces scallops, three ounces shrimp, ½ cup (cooked) fettuccine, 1½ cups veggies, sautéed in one teaspoon peanut oil.

Primavera ordered off some menus, of course, would blow your dietary regimen out the window. If it's a good restaurant, they'll cook it this way for you (easily done) and save you from clogging your arteries with sauce.

By the way, let's pretend Day Three is TGIF (Thank God It's Friday) and very mellow. You might want to try a white wine spritzer with your meal. More soda than wine, and quite refreshing.

EVENING SNACK (2-3 hours later)
1 small fruit
6 ounces protein drink
2 almonds

DAY FOUR:
BREAKFAST
½ cup (cooked) oatmeal
½ cup skim milk
4 ounces protein drink
4 ounces low-fat yogurt

LUNCH (2-3 hours later)
1 bowl chicken broth

Turkey sandwich made with 1 slice rye bread, 3 ounces turkey, and garnished with lettuce and veggies of choice
Small pear
6 cashews, unsalted

SEMI-MEAL (2-3 hours later)
1 ounce turkey sausage
1 kiwi *or* ½ cup applesauce

DINNER (2-3 hours later)
Chili made with three ounces ground turkey, ⅔ cup red beans, 1 cup tomatoes, ½ cup chopped onions and peppers, ⅓ cup oats, ½ cup salsa
Broccoli or other green vegetable as side dish

EVENING SNACK (2-3 hours later)
½ frozen banana
6 ounces protein drink
6 peanuts or 2 almonds

A REGIMEN FOR THE RAIL

Most Americans would love to have this guy's weight problem. But he or she represents a very substantial minority—people, mostly teens and young adults, who are thin and frail, all skin and bones, and need to put on some weight.

No, I am not going to recommend a diet of cheeseburgers, french fries and chocolate shakes. Even thin people develop heart disease if their arteries are jammed full of cholesterol. Neither am I going to recommend cookies and cake and soda pop. The idea is to add strong, lean tissue, not fat. Adding muscle means exercise and balanced nutrition—the same as it does for people of any body type.

The one day's menu plan shown below calls for a canned nutritional supplement. Many products are available from many manufacturers.

BREAKFAST
8 egg whites
1 cup of oatmeal, cooked with water
12 peanuts

MID-MORNING SNACK (2-3 hours later)
One 1,200-calorie gainer supplement (about three grams of fat and 10 to 12 grams of carbohydrate per eight grams of protein)

LUNCH (2-3 hours later)
½ pound roast beef (lean) on whole wheat bread
Green salad with tomato
1 tablespoon oil, plus vinegar
(flax or olive oil and apple cider vinegar would be my choice)
1 piece fruit

A good alternate lunch would be two whole four-ounce chicken breasts and a pasta salad, with a fruit.

MID-AFTERNOON SNACK (2-3 hours later)
One protein shake: two tablespoons egg-white protein powder (25 grams of fat-free protein), one cup 2 percent milk, one teaspoon peanut butter, one banana and three ice cubes, all mixed in blender.

DINNER (2-3 hours later)
2 five-ounce pieces of broiled or roasted chicken or fish
(whitefish, swordfish or tuna); *or* one 10-ounce steak
1 cup steamed broccoli
1 baked potato *or* corn on the cob
Spinach salad

MY OWN TRAINING DIET
This is typical of what I eat in, say, the last 12 weeks before a body-building competition. For most of this period, I'm in the gym for about 2 ½ hours of intensive training every day. So anybody who thinks you need to load up on milkshakes and cheeseburgers to get the job done is going to get a rude awakening.

BREAKFAST (5 a.m.)
10 egg whites

SECOND BREAKFAST (7:30 a.m.)
⅓ cup oatmeal, cooked in water, *or* four rice cakes.

MID-MORNING SNACK (10:30 a.m.)
1 broiled chicken breast and one frozen banana.

LUNCH (1 p.m.)
2 chicken breasts chopped up in a salad with one cup steamed green beans, one sliced tomato, alfalfa sprouts, one tablespoon flax oil, vinegar to taste, *or* two whole chicken breasts with a small pasta salad

MID-AFTERNOON SNACK (3 p.m.)
1 protein shake with two tablespoons egg white protein powder, one cup apple juice and three ice cubes, mixed in a blender

DINNER (6 p.m.)
1 six-ounce piece of broiled or roasted chicken or fish
½ cup steamed broccoli
1 baked potato *or* corn on the cob
Spinach salad

I get "full." Honest. Food is habit, habit, habit. What you see here is plenty of nutrition to keep an *extremely* active human body fueled, to maintain weight, to replenish muscle that is broken down in exercise. Scientifically speaking, those are the only reasons we eat.

Do I ever "reward" myself with special treats? Yes, of course. But never while I'm in training for a competition. Out of training is another story, and it's this: My basic nutritional regimen remains essentially as simple and lacking in sugars and salt and low in fat as what you see above. I'll reward myself on a Friday or Saturday night, or on a special occasion, or on a vacation trip. But I never fool myself into thinking that a thick slice of apple pie or a glass of Grand Marnier is a part of my daily diet. The human body wasn't built to run on that stuff, any more than your car was built to run on kerosene. Fuel it wrong, and the repair bill might be so high that you have no choice but to junk it.

14

Nutrition and Kids (Adults, Listen Up)

The biggest tragedy in our whole dismal fitness picture is our kids. As bad off as the adult population may be, tomorrow's American adults look worse. You don't even need to see obesity. All you need to do is look at the stuff our kids are eating, and you can take a time machine snapshot 20 years into the future. It's not pretty. I don't think "tragedy" overstates the case at all.

One study says that obesity among children aged 6 to 11 has increased 54 percent from 1970 to 1990. In the last decade of the century, this figure climbed even higher. Since obese kids are three times more likely to be obese adults, all those familiar remarks about "baby fat" are not only silly, they're lethal. Baby fat means there's a good chance you're getting an early glimpse of high blood pressure, high cholesterol and heart attack.

Those obese 6- to 11-year-olds see about 10,000 TV commercials a year for food. *This* is the way we communicate in modern America. Ten thousand messages, and not one of them says any of the things I've talked about here. Seen any commercials lately for unrefined, fibrous complex carbohydrates, packaged without sugar and salt? Seen any big-time jocks pulling down million-dollar endorsements to pitch apples or broccoli or omega-3 fatty acids? TV can be a marvelous medium. But mostly what it does to our kids is make them immobile, which is a crime, and train them to eat garbage, which makes TV a two-time felon. It's past time for parents, and any health-conscious adults, to get concerned about *this* kind of pornography, which has a well-documented effect on health.

A Harvard study projected that obesity among kids aged 12 to 17 increases by 2 percent for every weekly hour of television watched. A team at Stanford released a report recommending the obvious: a change in family lifestyle, including less TV time; more time together; more exercise—walking, cycling, hiking. Like the study suggests, you don't need a Nautilus or a health club membership to get exercise.

Many of our kids are getting into the yo-yo weight syndrome even before junior high. One study reported that nearly half of 9-year-olds and nearly 80 percent of 11-year-olds *had tried at least one fad diet!* Imagine! Only 9 years old, already with a weight problem, already doing exactly the wrong thing to turn it around.

Health is more than the absence of disease. It is a whole life attitude. It includes physical and mental well-being. More and more adults have decided that it's *chic* to be healthy. They exercise aerobically. They eat low-fat diets. They drink less alcohol. The tobacco smoke is clearing (but is still present, tragically, among teens). But too many people are left out. It's still a minority of the adult population that has a grasp on fitness. Even those who learn to think fit seldom pass it on to their children.

Teens can learn a healthy lifestyle, too, just like the enlightened adult minority. Teens can dare to be different, can defy the microwave and fast-food culture. They can take responsibility for their own health, can even become leaders in their group. If you are a parent, you have a serious responsibility to do all you can to help your kids down that path. If you're a teen, you need to evaluate your own habits and think about where you want to be a few years down the line. If you're smart enough, for example, to know that education will put you where you want to be, then you ought to be smart enough to know that it won't be anyplace worth being unless your body comes along with you.

Most teens don't carry typical middle-aged bodyfat around with them. But teens especially need to understand that being fit is more than having a certain percentage of bodyfat, or being able to lift a certain amount of weight, or to run a certain distance. It involves an attitude of discipline and self-respect and self-love. A truly fit person is concerned with both body and mind. When your attitude is "fit," then everything else will follow. And your self-confidence will peak.

Nobody, let alone a teenager who is subject to all that peer pressure and all those hormones, can wake up one morning and say, "OK, now I'm going to eat right." Small, gradual changes are the way to go. Too much change at once can turn your life upside down and leave you frustrated to the point that you give up. Small changes may seem slower, but they are *lasting* changes. If you read the basic nutritional information in this book, for example—*really* read it, and understand it—then you can start to *think* about your relationship with the cheeseburger and french fries. I mean, are there *drugs* in those things? Does your social standing depend on you living on them? Use that second lens to look at your food. Do you want to open up your stomach and pour all that fat in, time after time after time? Some serious modification of your relationship with the cheeseburger and fries would be a small change in your life, but—nutritionally speaking—it would be an important one.

Don't try to live on spinach. But start making some substitutes: low-fat cheese instead of regular, low-fat or nonfat yogurt instead of sour cream, a grilled chicken breast instead of a burger, grilled veggies instead of fries, a bottle of water instead of a cola, a walk down to the park instead of spacing out in front of TV or video games.

If you're a teen, you should know that the experts say we adults can't reach you with that kind of message—it's too cerebral. You kids are living too much for today. You feel too immortal. Maybe so. Maybe that's the best way of explaining how fortunate I was to get a big-time message of mortality when Crohn's hit me at age 15. Maybe if it weren't for the Crohn's, I'd be in line at the pork shop right now. I was *fortunate* to get sick, because it put me on the right path early on.

What happened to me at 15 was something that usually happens about 30 years later to many people, in one way or another. Your middle-aged body sends you a message that says: "I'm hurting." Often it's too late.

That's why I want to keep trying, in every way possible, to reach kids—and their parents—with my message.

Nutrition is where it all starts.

Part Three:
Sweat Equity

15

Starting at Square One

A lot of words get tossed around loosely when people talk about physical condition. "Fit," for example. And "active." As in: "He leads an active lifestyle and he's fit." Definitions of these words fall all over the map.

You know by now that my goal is to see an American society where most people are "fit"—particularly our kids, whose *un*fitness is a national scandal. Maybe your definition of "fit" is different than mine. For some, being fit means being able to get to and from the car without distress, or surviving a night out at the bars without an industrial-strength headache. I doubt that's your definition, or you wouldn't be reading this book. For sure, my definition of "fit" asks for a whole lot more than that.

I think the *average* person should have muscle tone instead of seriously excess body fat; should have arteries that are not threatened by a junk-food, fast-food diet; should have enough cardiovascular endurance to change a tire or walk 20 blocks without feeling like he's in the ninth round of a heavyweight bout; should be free of the chronic debilitating effects of tobacco use and alcohol abuse; should be a person whose self-image—and reality—portrays a body in motion, not slumped on a couch with pizza grease on the fingers and TV in the eyes.

I think the *average* person deserves, and needs, the confidence and self-esteem that come with achieving these minimal goals.

And I think that if the average American resembled that version of "being fit," then an amazing number of us would be taking it even further, to the next step. That's because fitness is as addictive as alcohol or tobacco. Except that fitness improves and lengthens life, instead of deteriorating and shortening it.

Nutrition can win you just a piece of that picture. You also *need* exercise to be the best that you can be. Everything from your work day to your sex life to your ability to play a piano to your ability to *think* clearly is enhanced by the full fitness package. We're talking about improving the quality of life on so many levels it boggles the mind. Any way you slice it, there's a very large empty space in the package if it doesn't include regular exercise.

The physical, mental and nutritional aspects of fitness are wrapped together so tightly that sometimes it's difficult to separate them. In this section, we're going to talk mainly about exercise. But let's back up a second and talk about this word "active." Here comes the mental part of the package again, because being active is really a state of mind, not of muscle.

You can't even begin an exercise program until you set the stage by taking control of your life in two ways: first, getting your nutritional life into the reality zone, and second, getting into an active state of mind. We've talked about the first. The second means that you don't regard your body as a sack of bricks to move from chair to chair through the day, and then to throw on the couch until it falls asleep at night. Being active means the opposite of being passive, in what is probably the most passive society that ever existed. We are out of control, but not in the sense of a car barreling down a mountain road at 120 mph. We're out of control in the sense of a car rusting in the backyard. We're sitting and waiting for the junkman.

And I've got news for you. When the body rusts, so does the mind. It's not just biceps and triceps that get put on hold when a couple hundred million human bodies vegetate in front of TV sets for hours on end. Whether you're watching "Batman" reruns or PBS, staring at the tube is *totally* passive. Even conversation stops. If you didn't have to blink and breathe, there would be no signs of human life. Maybe the best way to see this—like using that second lens on food—would be to climb behind your TV one evening and look back out the other way. Scary! Look at all those zombies!

I don't mean to say that TV is evil. In fact, I make part of my living appearing on TV. There's nothing evil about chocolate, either. But we don't lie on our backs all night and let some high-tech gizmo dump candy down our throats. (At least I haven't heard of that one yet.) I'm just using TV as the common denominator of how incredibly *passive* Americans have become. The ultra couch potato sits and consumes pictures and chips and dip. He doesn't *do* anything.

Nobody knows how many black-belt couch potatoes exist in the U.S. today. But it's pretty obvious that a huge percentage of the population holds at least a brown belt in vegetating.

Sure, we work hard all day. The surveys say we're working more hours than we did a generation ago. But the surveys also say we don't have much energy left to do anything else. We're *tired*. Nine or 10 hours of crunching numbers or peddling widgets and we just want to plop down and recuperate. If you're a numbers cruncher or a widget peddler, don't take offense, but the human *anatomy* was designed to handle a lot more than that. The human *mind* might not have been designed to handle that much tension and stress, but that's a different story. Your passive lifestyle, in fact, has got you in a vicious cycle. Your mind has tricked your body into telling you it's too tired to exercise, when *just the opposite is true*. Eat right, get up off that couch, and—in a reasonably short period of time—you'll have more energy for peddling widgets and crunching numbers than you've had in years. All that tension and stress will be more manageable, too.

It's time to get into training. First the mind, *then* the body. You push the "active" button with a brain cell, not a muscle. The ultra couch potato—or even the brown belt—can't jump up and start playing a tough hour of three-on-three basketball every night or run five miles every day. Those would be very decent ways of being active, but they would kill a couch potato. The ultra couch potato has slid back to Square One with his or her health. He or she must very carefully, very deliberately, take baby steps that progressively lead to increased physical activity.

It takes motivation to reverse years of bad habits and deterioration. That motivation has to come from within yourself. The main purpose of this book is motivational. But all that any book or speech, or personal training can do is light a spark. You have to keep the flame going yourself.

As far as I've been able to figure out in more than two decades of personal training, couch potatoes are people who don't really comprehend *why* they should become active. They don't really *believe* it'll make that much difference in their lives. "Sedentary" and "sedative" are dictionary cousins. Couch potatoes are too sedated by inactivity to focus on fitness. Many come to me for personal training only after a wakeup call in the form of a doctor's dire warning, a divorce, or some other trauma. *That* kind of motivation most people understand. So, couch potatoes, listen up. Here is a wakeup call *before* the trauma. Here are some reasons for getting into a new, active state of mind. Trust me; they're real.

1. Being active is a circuit breaker. It's a *vicious cycle* breaker. Physical activity eats up tension and frustration like a vacuum cleaner eats dirt. If everybody in the country took the active path all the way to fitness, the combined income of America's shrinks would drop 50 percent overnight.

2. Physical activity does good things to your body that will make you live longer. That's statistically speaking, of course. Mr. and Mrs. Muscle could get hit by a bus tomorrow, just like anybody else. Purging your body of excess fat and strengthening your cardiovascular system can't guarantee

that you won't get cancer or some other dread disease. But a fit body is far more likely to wind up on the positive side of the statistics. Studies prove that you can even dodge some hereditary bullets if you are fit.

3. You'll discover the meaning of quality time, and you'll have more of it.

4. You won't be afraid to look in the mirror. This reason alone is enough to deprive the therapists of a fair amount of business. It's also the least important reason for starting down the active path. But I have to tell you that appearance is absolutely the single biggest reason that people show up in health clubs or call on me for personal training. It's understandable, but it's wrong, wrong, wrong. Looking good is a tremendous fringe benefit to exercise. It's great. Can't beat the feeling. But it should be reason No. 4 for becoming active. If you don't get in tune with the other reasons, your whole exercise program—just like its motive—will be cosmetic, and it will fail. We'll talk a lot more about this later.

Those are four good reasons, by anybody's judgment, for becoming active. You can't buy the results, however, with anything but your own sweat equity.

If you are a true couch potato, the idea is *not* to put this book down right now, run out on the deck and start doing push-ups. Not unless you want, at best, to fail, or, at worst, to kill yourself. First, you must take steps to do something about your nutrition. That will get your brain seriously engaged in the fitness process. Then you must take a close look at just how physically passive your whole attitude has become toward "getting through the day." And then you must change that negative attitude into something a whole lot more positive.

Chances are just about 100 percent that you're pretty disgusted with yourself and ready for change. Otherwise, you wouldn't be reading these words. But running headlong into change will guarantee failure. Better to walk. Persistently, consistently, a little farther every day. Start by taking stock of just how *in*active you are, and how you got that way.

Partly, you are a victim of "progress." A century ago, getting through the day would guarantee that you would be fit, at least in terms of exercise. Things got done by hand and foot. Everything from washing yesterday's socks to getting down the road involved serious physical activity. People built and repaired things themselves. They planted and harvested without machinery. If they didn't walk, they had a horse and had to take care of it. Handling the reins for one round trip into town was as much exercise as two years' worth of power steering. In case you ever wondered how so many people managed to live into adulthood without modern medicine, that's probably the best explanation. Getting through the day burned lots of calories and involved plenty of aerobic (and usually anaerobic) exercise.

Now compare that with your world, which you have come to take for granted. Do I even need to paint the picture? How about just one symbol for the whole high-tech thing: your TV set's *remote control.* What an active person does is to *take remote control out of his or her life.* That is, ironically, the first step toward really, truly being in control. You don't have to go back to the 19th Century. Just get back into your body.

When you go to the mall, don't blow your cool when you can't park the air-conditioned buggy within two steps of the store. In fact, seek a parking space farther out. If you're meeting a friend, take a brisk walk together before you start shopping. When you go to a store on Level B, bypass the escalator and walk up the stairs. Back home, if you're addicted to music videos, don't just stare at the thing—get up and dance. If you're going to a convenience store two blocks away, walk. If you're going to visit a friend 10 blocks away, ride a bike. Don't gripe because the kid hasn't gotten home to take out the garbage; do it yourself. Instead of watching some rerun, take care of a household chore you've been putting off. These are relatively painless steps, even for the most confirmed couch potato. Take them all, a few more each day.

In the process, you'll start to get your mind in tune with your body, just like you developed that second lens for looking at food. You'll start to remember that you *do* have a body, the one all those remote controls made you forget.

This is a wondrous, complex machine you live within—far more so than all the electronic toys that isolate your mind and muscles from the real world. You have about 600 muscles, in fact, and 100 million muscle fibers. Every movement you make—running two miles or blinking an eye or moving your food through the digestive tract—is done by muscles. In the couch potato state of mind, we forget all that. In the fit state of mind, we can never forget. It's the couch potato who performs some simple task and then the next day moans: "Man, I used some muscles I didn't even know I had."

That's not just a cliché. It's true for millions of Americans. They prefer to let their muscles remain anonymous. If they climb a tree for the first time in 20 years or go on a hike while vacationing at the Grand Canyon, the anonymity disappears suddenly and painfully. If a couch potato gets a flat tire that takes him out of his 65 m.p.h. cocoon to do some manual repair for the first time in 10 years, he's liable to do a macho tire change and pop a muscle. These kinds of injuries—on the job or in day-to-day living—are enough reason to take fitness seriously. You can't assume that your body will continue moving, in its complex ways, as long as you live in it. When it starts creaking like a 120,000-mile car, you'll be trying to fix it a day late and a dollar short.

I believe the greatest secret in making this attitude shift is to make your mind work *for* you instead of against you. You do this by constantly thinking positively—even if what you're thinking about is negative, like 50 pounds of excess fat. And how do you do this? By setting goals. Goals are not ideals. Ideals are something way down the road. Maybe you'll get there someday. Goals are things you can attain today, tomorrow, next week, next month, this year. They are realistic. You can reach them and check them off your list, and that's why you'll succeed. Instead of failing, you'll meet one goal, and then set out for the next one. That's why it's not trivial and not silly to make walking farther from your car a goal when you go to the mall tomorrow. It's going to be a whole lot of days before you can check "minus 50 pounds" off your list of long-term goals.

Couch potatoes, believe me. Many readers who have advanced far, far past this chapter in their personal fitness regimen know exactly what I'm talking about. They've been there. *Don't think you're alone.* You are suffering the national disease. You're no Davy Crockett blazing a new trail away from fatigue and low self-esteem. That's a positive in itself. You're not the first person to let your body slide so far. Recognize that fact. Instead of letting your current condition be a negative, dragging you even further down, take stock, set realistic goals and move forward—knowing you have lots of company. You're not exactly coming out of the closet. Everybody close to you knows you're in there.

With a sound nutrition regimen and an active state of mind, it won't be long before you'll be seeking exercise goals a little more stiff than walking a few blocks to pick up the Sunday paper. If you're only a partial couch potato, you're already set for an introductory conditioning program. In either case, this is a good place to give you a warning/reminder. *Get a physical exam.*

Years of inactivity have put your body on course for a shock. A little soreness is nothing to worry about. A heart attack is. Before you start a program, get a checkup (which you're probably overdue for anyway) and tell your doctor what you're about to do. Ask him or her specifically if you have any abnormal limitations in exercising. While you're at it, tell him that you're on a new, balanced nutrition regimen, and that you intend to stay on it the rest of your life. His diagnosis for your whole plan probably will be: "It's about time."

16

Plain and Simple —
The Basics of Muscle Conditioning

Maybe it's just human nature. Maybe it's just the American way in the age of high tech. But so often when we're tackling a problem, we do two things: first, we run out and buy a gadget to do the job, and second, we make it much more complicated than it has to be.

Take a look at a suburban two-car garage. What's in there, two cars? No. Gadgets. Here's a $500 snow shovel that will scoop the white stuff up off the sidewalk and spit it on the lawn. Here's a $2,500 lawn mower you can ride on. Here's a $150 rake that *blows* leaves into a pile. Here's the invention of the century: a fishing line attached to an internal combustion engine (it whacks weeds). I shouldn't have to point out that every one of those gadgets is designed to keep your muscles anonymous. Household gadgets and being active usually aren't a good match.

So it goes when we decide to start exercising—to take those first small steps toward conditioning. Too many people think the only way to get the job done is to run out and buy a gadget. Some of these exercise gadgets cost a *lot* of money. And most of them are complicated, even if they look like a piece of Scandinavian furniture. You have to make adjustments to do different exercises. While you fiddle around with the machine, you lose "the pump," that warm glow of a workout in progress that begs you to keep going *now*.

You *can* condition yourself on these in-home universal machines. But my experience has been that many people find them too intimidating. Or, like a kitchen gadget that winds up rusting in the back of a drawer, people get bored with them. When somebody asks me about them, my usual response is something like: "You're probably better off to take your five grand, go back to the basics, spread the money over a couple of years and hire a professional to come in and be your personal trainer." I don't say that to drum up business, but because it's true.

Fitness is best approached plain and simple. That's especially important at Square One, when you're not trying to win a Mr. Universe or a North American swimming title or a triathlon. All you want is to slim down, tone up and make your body start working for you instead of against you. You're trying to stay in an active state of mind, in touch with your body. The last thing you want to do is to go out and buy a high-tech gadget. Every corner of your brain associates gadgets with something being done *for* you. Fitness is 100 percent something you are going to do for yourself.

Make it simple. Make it fun.

Let me tell you, for example, about three plain and simple—and cheap— ways to give yourself a workout. The first one doesn't cost you a dime. The second one uses a dime-store piece of equipment that probably is sitting in your basement or attic. The third one uses a piece of equipment you can buy at the drugstore for less than $5. All three are fun. All three can easily be done by recovering couch potatoes who have *never* worked out. But at least two of them are also practiced regularly by champion athletes. All can be done in the privacy of your own home—or in a motel room while on a sales trip or on vacation. These are workouts that remind me, in the best of ways, of when I was getting started back in my grandmother's basement in Brooklyn.

The first workout method is incredibly simple, despite its imposing name: *manual resistance training*. It sounds so formal, so heavy, so macho. But it's the least formal thing you ever heard of. As for macho, well, about all you need for equipment are a towel and a broomstick. No dumbbells, no barbells, no iron weights. I've done this on the TV talk shows. Here comes a guy (me) who looks like he's been training for years with megaweights, and he's running around the stage with a towel and a broomstick and another piece of equipment that I'll mention in a minute. Hey, anything to get people thinking fitness.

Before we even get to the towel and broomstick, you have to understand that there's a substitute for everything. Take two cans of tomato juice, for example, or whatever canned goods you have handy. Didn't know you had dumbbells on the shelf, did you? Start walking rapidly in place, or jogging. Then pick up your "dumbbells," and hold them palms up with your arms straight down at your sides. Then, keeping your upper arms straight downward, raise one can up to your shoulder, then straight back down. While your left forearm is going down, use your right forearm to bring the other can up. You are now doing alternate dumbbell curls. First you did a little aerobics with your walking or jogging, then you did some resistance work with the cans. And you're starting to feel a nice burn.

You say you're too shy or embarrassed to go to the gym, at least not yet? Well, who's going to tell on you? The cat? He may be a little confused at all this activity, but he won't talk.

Anyway, courtesy of a couple of cans and your own creativity, you're now getting a little taste of "the pump." Take a 30- to 60-second rest while shaking out your arms. Then use the cans again, this time in a lateral movement, with your arms starting at your sides and rising—together and slightly bent—to about ear height. Do 10 or 15 of these. Then take that 30- to 60-second rest, which is something you'll be doing between exercises even if you wind up pumping iron in the fanciest gym. Then do alternate front laterals—raising one arm at a time in a forward motion.

Now you're warmed up. We'll come right back to manual resistance training, but let's go for a minute to that other piece of equipment in your basement or attic. This is the one that I'm not aware of any champion athletes using, but believe me, it's one terrific form of exercise. We're talking *hula hoop.* This is one fad that never should have died.

Put on some music on the stereo or TV. Your cat is really going to laugh at this one, but who cares? Slip that old hoop over your head and start twisting. In case you forgot, the object is to keep the hoop above your waist. It's going to fall on the floor, guaranteed. Pick it up and twist harder. This is *very* tiring stuff. You are working your abdominals, your obliques, your intracostals, your back. If you are a true couch potato, tomorrow you're going to feel like you were hit by a sledgehammer—and you'll work it right back out. And if you're feeling silly at first, don't forget: *I* did this on TV and survived.

Seriously, the hula hoop is first-class exercise. In a small way, it's a version of the cross-training (aerobic and anaerobic) that we'll talk about later. Don't try to do the hula hoop all afternoon first time out. In fact, after taking a couple of minutes to remember how to keep the hoop up, twist your way vigorously through maybe just one song—about three minutes. You ought to be keeping a fitness diary, or log. Today you can write down something like: "Hoop: one song. Try two songs next time."

Now, back to manual resistance training—with a nice sweat worked up.

As with any kind of exercise, you'll get the best results if you have a training partner. So why not get your spouse, a friend, or a parent—or a grandparent—involved? He or she can use the workout, and you can use the physical resistance and the moral support.

Take the bath towel and do some pulls. Remember that your partner's actions are a mirror image of your own. Whatever movements you make, whatever muscles you work, will be done on the opposite side of your partner's body.

Roll the towel up lengthwise, so it's like one long, thick rope. You grasp one end, your partner the other. Plant your left foot forward, with the left side of your body turned toward your partner, towel held firmly at stomach level, right hand in back and left hand forward. Your partner has reversed all that, and is planted on the other side of the towel. Like the name of the exercise says, you *pull*. Pull, breathe, relax, stretch while your partner pulls back; then repeat. Do the exercise to failure—when you start to feel a muscle burn; then reverse positions and do it again. You don't know what it means yet, but what you are doing is kind of a mini-version of super-sets for your biceps and your back. Pull for biceps; stretch for back.

Now face each other and hold the towel horizontally. You grasp it, wide grip, palms under. Curl up. Meanwhile, your partner, palms above the towel with a narrow grip, pushes downward. Curl, breathe, relax. Do a vigorous set of 10. Take your 30- to 60-second rest, then reverse positions and repeat the exercise. Curling up, you're working your biceps; pushing down, you're working your triceps.

You see the concept. You can clone almost any gym exercise as long as there's resistance. Weight training is resistance training, with iron supplying the resistance. Manual resistance is very light training, and you cannot build a Mr. Universe body—or even a Mr. Saskatchewan—by doing manual resistance. You *can*, however, burn calories and tone muscle. It is fitness plain and simple. In a way, manual resistance was made for the beginner. A 120-pound barbell will supply 120 pounds of resistance from now until doomsday. When a lifter tires, he's stuck. In manual resistance training, when you—or your partner—tires, there is less resistance.

You can tie a towel to a door or a heavy piece of furniture. If you've got a *long* towel, you can stand on one end. It's best, however, to have a partner. If you have a partner and a broomstick, you can even replicate some specific weight-training exercises. Still plain and simple. And fun.

You lie on the floor, for example, grasp the broomstick shoulder-width like a barbell and push upward—breathing out at the hardest part of the exercise. It's hard because your partner, standing above, is grasping the stick and providing downward resistance. Now you're doing bench presses with no bench and no weights. All of the principles of weight resistance training—repetitions, breathing, rest, etc., which we'll talk about later—apply to these simple broomstick exercises. Remember, muscle starts to atrophy after *12 hours* of inactivity. You can't build masses of muscle doing manual resistance training, but if you have been inactive for, say, *12 years,* then you *will* build muscle with that broomstick, that hula hoop and that towel.

Now here's that third piece of equipment I mentioned. It's called the Dynaband. As you've seen, I'm not into touting specific brand names in this book, but this little jewel is something special. You can buy the Dynaband at most chain drugstores for less than $5. They look something like a bicycle tire inner tube and they come in three different colors, for three different degrees of resistance.

Couch potatoes, kids, grandparents and stay-at-home-spouses can make good use of the Dynaband, and have fun while they're at it. Pro body-builders use them to warm up backstage at competitions, or for a mini-workout when they can't get to a gym. I've got an old picture of Schwarzenegger and Sergio Olivia, a couple of champions, warming up together with Dynabands. I use the Dynaband myself, often.

Portable? Stick it in the corner of a briefcase and you've got a gym wherever you go. There's never an excuse for not working out.

Put it under your foot and do curls for your biceps. Do leg pulls for your outer thighs. Do arm pulls for your chest and shoulders. It's excellent manual resistance conditioning, as good as you can get without a partner. And, of course, you can do a Dynaband workout with a partner, too.

So what's the real point of talking about towels and broomsticks and drugstore equipment that looks like an inner tube? Creativity. Fun. Lack of intimidation. A door to the active path that's open to anyone. No matter how far out of shape they are. No matter how embarrassed they are. No matter how little money they have. No matter how little time they have. Once you become *active*—remember, it's a state of mind—you'll understand that exercise, and all its rewards, is right there for the taking. Instant gratification without spending big bucks.

The inactive person goes down to the lake on a Saturday afternoon and looks at the water. The active person—even if he can't swim from here to the dining room—discovers that it's incredible exercise to walk or jog in knee-deep water. It burns calories and is tremendous for the legs.

The inactive person watches America's Team on TV while a hired kid does the yard. The active person cuts the grass and whacks the weeds himself. He wears a hat, drinks plenty of fluids and burns 550 calories an hour. He's in tune with his body, and he knows that he's doing more than using up an hour's time and making his neighbors happy.

I *love* the gym. Once you reach a certain plateau of fitness, there are things you can do in the gym that you can't do anywhere else. I work out on a half-million dollars' worth of equipment, and it pays off. But I also work out with my Dynaband. And one of the best exercises I do, every morning at home, is half push-ups with my feet on the bed. Zero equipment, unless you count the bedroom rug.

A lot of this, of course, goes back to my grandmother's basement. And to Julie's gym, where champions were born but no awards were won for interior design. Plain and simple.

One day—maybe even right now—you might be ready for the gym. But it's not the only place to get exercise. And it doesn't have to cost a dime.

17

You Gotta Have Heart —
The Basics about Cardiovascular Conditioning

Let's go back to that average out-of-shape driver whose air-conditioned cocoon blows a tire on the freeway. The suit coat comes off, the sleeves get rolled up, the jack comes out of the trunk. In a few minutes, our friend is going to get a double whammy. He is going to discover that he is seriously lacking in both kinds of fitness—endurance and strength.

Soon after lugging the spare out of the trunk and squatting down to yank on the lug wrench, he's sucking wind. Aerobically speaking, his cardiovascular endurance is about equal to the Happy 40th Birthday balloon that has been hanging around—barely—for a couple of weeks.

Then, trying to twist the fifth lug nut, he finds that right at the moment he probably couldn't twist the top off a pop bottle. His *strength*—something built up anaerobically through resistance against muscle, whether by weights pumped in the gym or by boxes unloaded from a truck—is non-existent.

There, in a graphic nutshell, you see some obvious reasons for conditioning your body along both fitness paths. Aerobics training and resistance training are two entirely different animals, but in the real world they go together like country and western. (Remember, we don't talk ham and eggs on our new dietary regimen.) Aerobics and anaerobics. Endurance and strength. Work on them both in a conditioning program and you can say that you're into "cross-training."

Imagine, for example, that you have worked yourself up to a three-day-a-week regimen—in your own basement—of 20 minutes of jump rope or hula hoop (aerobics), followed by a Dynaband routine (anaerobics). That would make you as solidly into cross-training as if you had a personal trainer and access to a million-dollar gym.

For starters, you need to know something about aerobics.

If you really are at a starting point, losing fat is undoubtedly one of your goals. Aerobic exercise is the fat-burning king. You could go dancing with your spouse and—assuming you stayed on your feet and the tempo stayed up—you could boogie off 600 calories in a very aerobic evening. An hour of working your way through a weight-lifting routine—even if you power-lifted the Empire State Building—would burn off practically zilch.

The fat-burning qualities of aerobics is an attention-getter for couch potatoes (see Chapter 11). But the real reason for pursuing aerobic fitness is what it does for the heart. Aerobics, in fact, strengthens the entire cardiovascular system. More oxygen gets to the cells that need it, and it becomes easier for your heart to get it there. An aerobically fit individual's heart beats about *17 million* fewer times in the course of a year. You don't need to be a physiologist to understand what that means.

In terms of performance, the big fringe benefit is endurance. We've got quite an endurance range in this crazy modern world where exercise is something we have to schedule into our lives. The air-sucking tire changer, for example, might be a salesman who works right across the desk from a marathoner. Both of them good people, both of them kind to their spouses and children, both of them wearing $1,000 suits, both of them driving big new cars. But one of them can run 26 miles and one of them can't change a tire. The wild thing is that I'm not exaggerating the comparison for effect. You'll find that exact Mutt and Jeff duo in the real world, in almost any office.

So what does Mutt have to do to get into some kind of cardiovascular reality zone, besides taking remote controls out of his life? Specifically, he should exercise aerobically three or four days a week, keeping his heart at its ideal target rate for at least 20 to 30 minutes. Here's what that's about.

Put two fingers on your wrist and take a pulse for 10 seconds. Multiply by six. That's your *resting heart rate.*

If you're a woman or an out-of-shape man, subtract your age from 220. If you're a man in very fit condition, subtract half your age from 205. That's a calculation of your *maximum heart rate.*

To get your *ideal target rate* for aerobic exercise, calculate 60 to 70 percent of your maximum rate.

An aerobic exercise program means that you take your heart to its ideal target rate, sustain it there for a certain period of time, and do the workout a certain number of times per week. Different authorities suggest slightly different numbers for all those variables. The ones I follow are the American Heart Association (the ideal target rate of 60 to 70 percent of

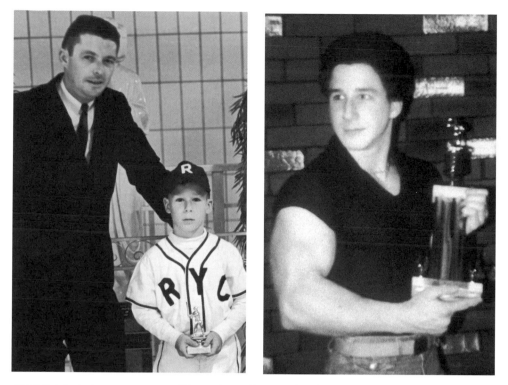

While Dad was pretty proud of my "Peewee League" trophy (left), he was even more excited when I won my first bodybuilding award (right). It was for 5th place in Armstrong County, PA.

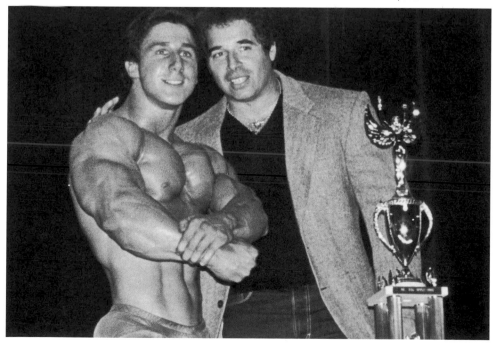

I credit Julie Levine (pictured with me above at the Mr. New York contest) for taking a self-trained basement weightlifter and turning him into a professional bodybuilder.

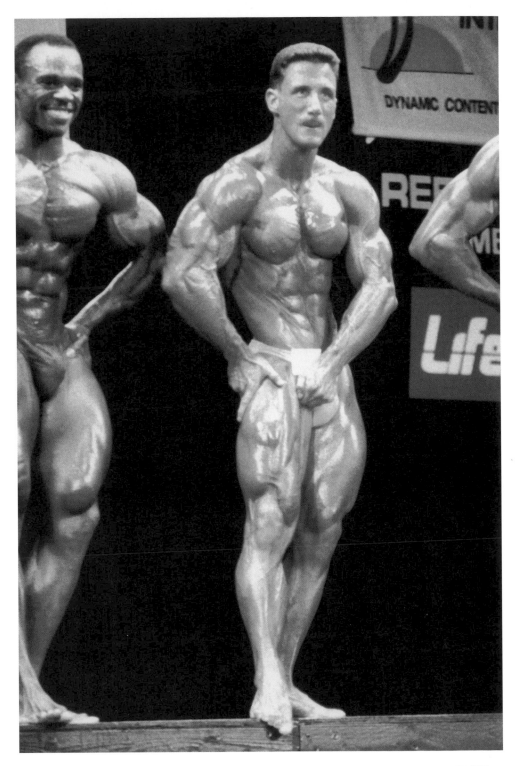

I FIRST GOT INTO THE SPORT OF BODYBUILDING TO SAVE MY LIFE AND ENDED UP TAKING IT TO THE HIGHEST LEVEL OF COMPETITION. HERE'S ME STRIKING THE WINNING POSE AT A MR. WORLD EVENT.

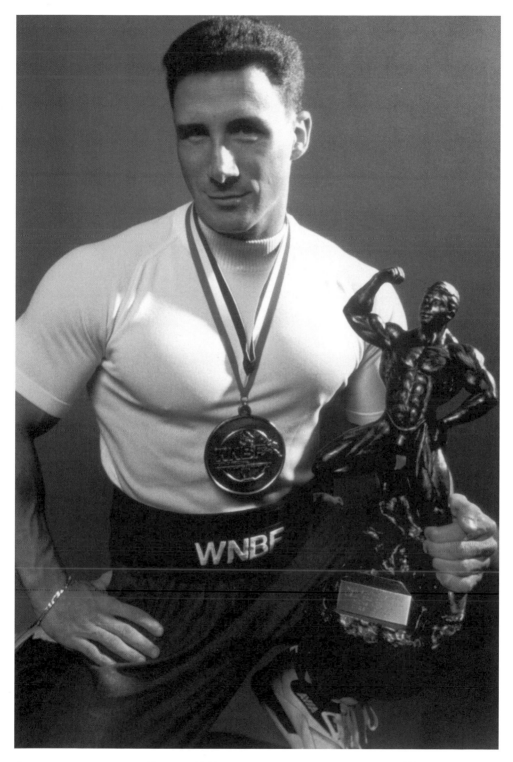

I came out of retirement in November 1991 and took the first place trophy in the NGA regional USA. I went on to win a medal by finishing 4th in the World Cup.

CINDY — WHO CAN OUTRUN ME BY SEVERAL MILES — IS NO SLOUCH IN THE GYM HERSELF. WE GRACED THE COVER OF THE FEBRUARY 1992 ISSUE OF *NATURAL PHYSIQUE* MAGAZINE.

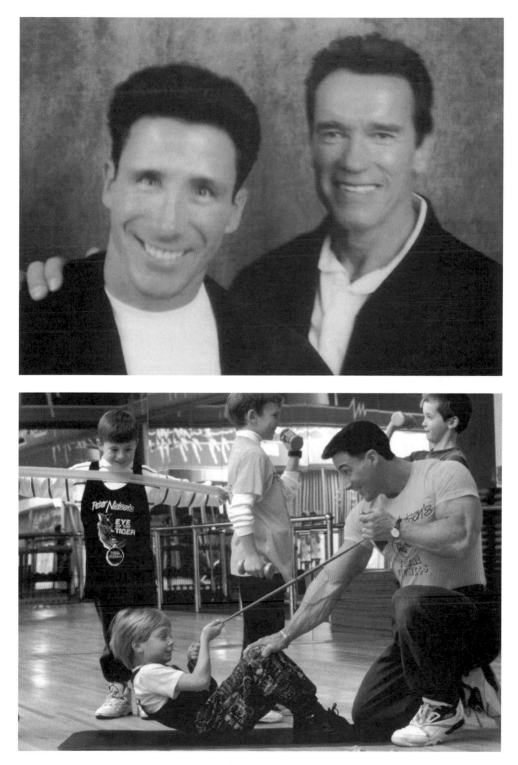

It's always a pleasure to run into Arnold Schwarzenegger (above) at health conferences, but I get even more enjoyment from teaching kids about my message of health, fitness and lifestyle.

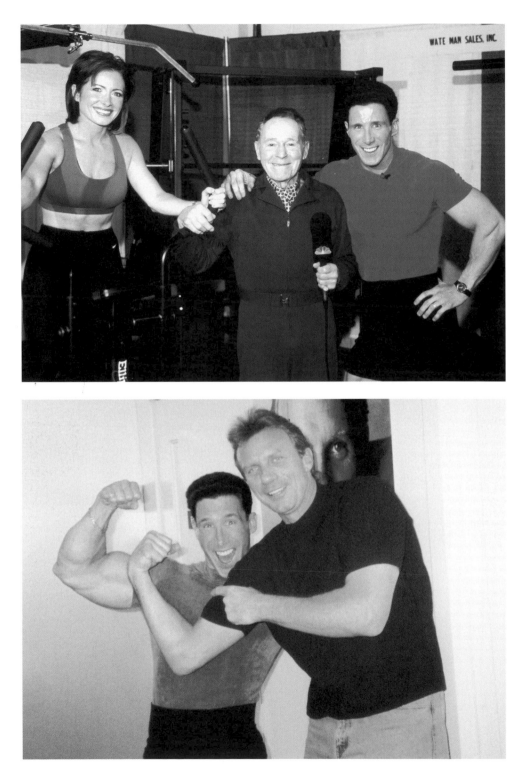

JACK LaLANNE (TOP CENTER) SUMS UP MUCH OF WHAT I'VE ALWAYS WANTED TO BE. AND JOE MONTANA (ABOVE) IS A HERO TO MANY FOOTBALL FANS. I THANK THEM BOTH FOR THEIR KIND WORDS ABOUT ME AND MY BOOK.

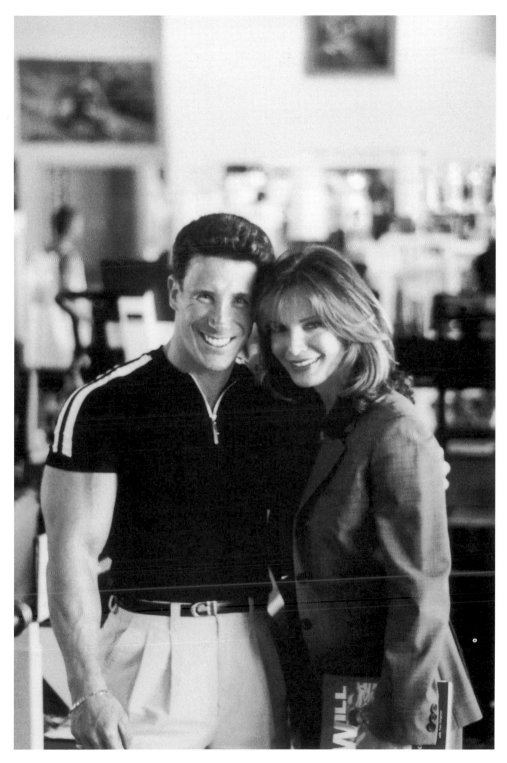

JACLYN SMITH STOPPED BY MY GYM TO TAPE A SEGMENT OF PETER'S PRINCIPLES FOR NBC. AND, OF COURSE, SHE HAS A COPY OF THE FIRST EDITION OF WILL OF IRON.

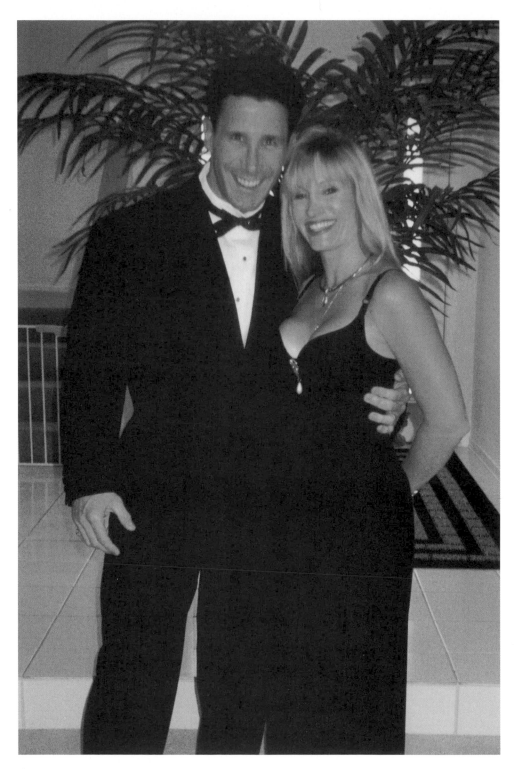

GETTING THROUGH MY ILLNESS SHOWED ME THAT I WANT MORE TIME WITH MY FAMILY — EVERY DAY. AND AFTER A HARD DAY AT WORK, IT'S NICE TO TAKE MY BETTER HALF OUT FOR A NIGHT ON THE TOWN.

maximum) and the Institute for Aerobic Research (four times a week, 20 minutes per session; or three times a week, 30 minutes a session).

What's going on while you exercise aerobically? Your blood becomes more oxygen-rich, and at the same time removes more carbon dioxide from all your body's cells after delivering the oxygen. Your muscle cells become more efficient at processing oxygen and eliminating lactic acid (meaning you won't have the lactic acid soreness that follows anaerobic exercise). Your blood vessels become more flexible, so your heart is less taxed. Lung capacity increases. Your heart, itself a muscle, becomes better supplied with blood and grows stronger. Your supply of HDL (good) cholesterol increases, while the supply of LDL (bad cholesterol) decreases.

And then there's your resting heart rate. An unconditioned person's heart may beat as much as 80 times a minute *at rest*. A person with good cardiovascular fitness will have a resting heart rate of 45 to 50 beats a minute. A superbly conditioned endurance athlete might have a resting rate in the range of 40 beats a minute.

Meanwhile, as we said when discussing nutrition, your basal metabolism rate stays higher even *after* aerobic exercise. So there you sit, burning calories and asking less of your heart. The beer commercials have it all wrong. It doesn't get any better than *this*.

If you work out too hard, you cross that anaerobic threshold. The heart loses all that efficiency in delivering oxygen and carting away carbon dioxide. You are no longer endurance training, and you will—in fact—have no endurance. You'll slow down, or quit, from exhaustion.

As your cardiovascular system becomes more fit, your anaerobic threshold will rise. More fit individuals can train at 75 to 80 percent of their maximum heart rate. Exceptionally fit individuals might even be able to train aerobically above 80 percent. Physiologists can determine your threshold with a treadmill test. The two-finger pulse check and the 60 to 70 percent target rate will work fine for starters. It's important to keep tab of your pulse, though, because you don't want to work yourself beyond the anaerobic threshold. It's not a health-threatening line if you cross it; but it will mean a quick end to the aerobic effect, and a quick end to your workout. (If you're chapter-skipping, by the way, we'll remind you that you should get a physical exam before launching any fitness regimen after a long period of inactivity.)

You can do specific aerobic exercises in the gym, or in your living room. But *any* exercise that takes your heart to its ideal target rate, sustains it and doesn't cross the anaerobic threshold is aerobic exercise. A long, brisk walk in your Levi's, bringing your dog along for *his* exercise, is just as aerobic as running in place in designer tights while watching a $50 exercise tape.

Jogging is one of the all-time great aerobic exercises. Many sports and activities, as we'll see in a minute, spill over—in varying degrees—to that gray area of cross-training.

Anaerobic exercise (literally "without oxygen") involves a quick, maximum thrust of energy. Aerobic exercise is a sustained, plodding activity in which the heart is stoking up the body with oxygen and burning up energy. Anaerobic exercise is a burst of effort that cannot possibly be sustained. Sprinting is anaerobic. Jogging is aerobic. Doing 10 bench presses with a heavy barbell is anaerobic. Dancing like a kid through your living room is aerobic. When you provide *resistance* against the sustained burst of effort, you are building muscle. Resistance is relative. Two hundred pounds of iron disks, for example, is stone cold resistance. The sets of exercises that make up a weightlifting routine are pure anaerobic resistance training. Don't tell a sprinter, however, that he is encountering no resistance when he drives off the starting blocks and pushes his body forward for 50 incredibly tense meters, trying to improve his time by a few hundredths of a second. His thighs will tell him there is resistance. (You could set a world dash record, by the way, without getting in a lick of aerobic exercise; at least not in the running of the race.)

A swimmer doing laps in relatively leisurely fashion is getting a first-class aerobic workout. A swimmer dashing a lap is not exercising aerobically. He is, however, encountering real resistance from the water with every stroke. Put a pair of those floppy leather mitts on his hands and he'd be meeting resistance equal to a modest dumbbell.

Cross-country skiing is excellent aerobic exercise. Ask anybody who has tried it about the uphills, though. Plenty of resistance there.

So there is haphazard cross-training in most any recreational sport that involves sustained physical exertion and bursts of maximum effort. It is, however, just that: haphazard. And generally not very symmetrical. The thighs of a speed skater would be one good example. You generally can get aerobically fit by "going out to play." Anaerobic conditioning is more tricky. A full-body resistance training program is the only way to systematically strengthen muscles in all the body parts. For that matter, specific resistance exercises are the best way to strengthen any particular muscles that need extra work. That's why athletes from football, basketball, hockey— dozens of entirely different sports—head to the gym for conditioning.

An inactive person most definitely wants to get his or her conditioning program started with aerobics. Burn that fat. Strengthen that heart. Get that BMR raised. The benefits are all pretty obvious. Aerobics is the *core* of turning a flabby society into a fit society. It *will* tone muscle. Strength can be built in various individual and team sports. If the whole country were riding bicycles and rowing and playing soccer, I'd be deliriously happy. But it should be no great surprise to learn that I believe almost anyone can benefit from weight training, if they choose to try it. Most people would rather cut the grass or clean out the cat's litter box. I think an amazing number would change their minds if they got into lifting.

What are the benefits?

First of all, if you're looking to build muscle, the weight room is the best place to be. No other game or sport that I know of directs work exactly to the muscles that need it, parcels out the work within a brief period of time and puts you entirely in command of what happens to your body. We've come a long way just within my lifetime in terms of working a weight program into a total fitness concept. Instead of going into the gym and jerking macho poundage a few reps at a time, we warm up and cool down aerobically. The power-lifting branch of the sport still measures life by how many pounds they can put in the air, but most of us think in terms of overall strength, endurance and muscle tone.

Which leads us to the cosmetic fringe benefit. That applies to aerobics as well, of course, because cosmetic step one is to shed the fat. Cosmetic step two—the one that crosses the T's and dots the I's—is to replace the fat with some solid lean tissue. I keep saying this is the least important reason to be fit. But we do live in a Vogue and GQ world. The pressures to look our best are intense. Besides, firming up the body does wonders for mental health. It's a whole lot healthier and cheaper than plastic surgery. And it will give an excuse—a necessity—for buying some new clothes.

Back on a more important vein, don't let that buzzword "strength" get in the way of your thinking. "Strength" doesn't mean you're a musclehead. It takes strength to carry a briefcase and a sample kit to a dozen appointments a day. It takes strength to clean house. Our friend discovered it takes strength to change a tire. It takes strength *to get up out of a chair.* Strength is a part of everyday life. Your cardiovascular system *and* your muscles deteriorate every day you're inactive. Every *year* that you're inactive, the toll gets more serious. Until finally, a minor little unfamiliar movement pops a muscle or a tendon somewhere. Aches and pains often are a body's way of saying: "I've got no strength." Weight training is a good way to answer: "Here you are."

If you already are an active person, if you are an athlete, that's all the more reason to become a lifter. I've trained pro athletes from every type of sport. All of them need specific strengths, and there's a way of improving performance in any sport through a specific weight program. A football linebacker basically needs to be able to push cattle around. A basketball player needs to protect and improve his already incredible leaping ability.

Hockey players fly down the ice, but they need tremendous upper body strength to win those shoving matches in the corners. I trained a college quarterback known for his agility and flexibility. He was obviously not interested in bulking up with a heavy-duty anaerobic program. But he needed to keep his legs strong, and a program of supersets increased his endurance.

In other words, weight training—for all this talk about muscle—is meant to help you get to the point where you don't even have to *think* about your muscles. It's a way of getting ready for life's combat, whatever that might be: knocking down a lineman, changing a tire, cleaning a house, rehabilitating an injury. Weights—and other forms of resistance training—are a piece of overall fitness and well-being. Some bodybuilders become obsessed with it, for sure. But have you talked to any golfers lately? You tell me which is the healthier obsession: tapping a little white ball or building muscle?

The fact is, most fit people that I know in daily life away from the gym play racquetball or swim or play tennis. They walk a lot. What resistance training they do is with Dynabands and 10-pound dumbbells. They are at an advanced state of aerobic fitness, and that's where they want to be.

That's fine. Weights aren't for everyone.

But as you design a new lifetime nutrition and exercise path, kick a few tires. You don't buy a new car without checking out all the models and options, and your body is a lot more important than a new car. A health club isn't a bad place to start, even if you ultimately take your act back out on the road. A good club offers both aerobic and anaerobic options and has qualified staff to help you choose a path that works for you. A bad club will burn your money and waste your time.

If you can afford it, if you find the idea of going to a club to be a motivating factor for fitness, and if you want to test the various waters, here's a checklist of factors for choosing a club. Some of them may seem obvious, but I've seen every one of them turn out to be the difference between a good and bad choice.

- Is the club open when workouts will fit your schedule? If so, find out whether it has kept those hours long enough to suggest they won't change next month.

- Is it near your home or office? Ten miles might not seem like much in your initial enthusiasm. But what about two months from now when you're dragging after a hard day and it's time for your workout?

- What can you afford? Cost of membership varies widely. Some clubs have family plans at reduced rates. Many offer occasional specials for new members. If this is strictly a test drive, availability of a short-term membership might be a big factor.

- What about general upkeep? Are weight machines in good working order? Are the locker rooms clean? Take a good look around the place. If you don't want to be there today, you certainly won't want to be there in six weeks.

- How well-equipped is the club? Are there plenty of aerobics devices, such as treadmills, bikes, and studios for aerobics, spinning, or kickboxing? Is the floor of the aerobics studio shock-compensated? Is there an adequate number of strength developing devices, including weight machines and free weights? Anywhere you have to wait for time with a device is a bad place to work out. You don't want to live there. You want to get in, have an intense training session, and get out.

- Is there at least one exercise physiologist on staff who is certified by the American College of Sports Medicine? It's important to have someone on hand who knows how to instruct you instead of just looking pretty.

- Are staff members certified in CPR? That's not meant to scare you. It's just another little sign that management is on its toes.

- Does it offer programs that interest you? Some clubs, for example, emphasize racquet sports. If you don't play racquet sports, you won't much care. The same applies to a swimming pool, which can account for a big piece of your membership fee.

- Are you looking for a place to meet friends, as well as to exercise? If so, does it offer a place for socializing?

- How much individual attention will you get? Is personal training offered? Will an exercise program be customized for your needs? Will it cost extra?

- Which items—massage, manicure, personal training, tanning, dining facilities, juice bar, etc.—are *a la carte* and which come with the club?

- Do you know someone who is already a member? If so, ask him or her to rate the club. If you're lucky enough to have this option, it's one of the best barometers.

• Beware of gyms staffed by overly sculptured employees who are too busy staring at their own reflections in the mirror to help you find your way around. That isn't a physique; that's a musclehead.

• Visit several clubs and ask for a tour. Make all of your visits on a day and at a time when you would be likely to be working out. It'll give you a true sense of traffic. The same club that looks uncrowded at 10 a.m. might be a zoo at 5:30 p.m.—after work, and just when you'd normally be showing up.

• Don't join any club without first trying out the facilities. Many will let you do so free of charge, at least for one visit. If not, it's worth paying the one-time rate.

Some people have the discipline and enough knowledge or self-study prowess to get a genuine conditioning program up and running at home, on their own. Some people don't. If you fall in the latter group, don't be one of the thousands of people who don't try a club because they're embarrassed by their flabby bodies. This is where shopping around and kicking tires becomes vitally important. Clubs have diverse clientele just like bars and restaurants. You don't, obviously, want to be in a power-lifters' gym. But you also don't want to be in a pleasant, attractive room where the emphasis is on socializing rather than fitness. Look and you'll find a place that meets a happy medium.

And, trust me, half the people in the place were wary, if not terrified, the first time they showed up for a workout. That feeling will disappear, along with the flab and the aches and pains.

18

Anatomy of a Workout

They don't call it a "routine" for nothing. An exercise program requires discipline of structure. Patterns in choosing the exercises themselves. Safety precautions. Warmup and cooldown. When you're doing the actual work, you're doing *repetitions,* or reps.

It all sounds so dreary. To be honest, on some days, it *can* be dreary. Being fit doesn't mean you're emotionless, or that your biorhythms somehow hum into a single, glowing groove. One day you'll go into the gym or into the basement full of physical and mental energy. Another day, you'll be drained. It could be for a thousand reasons. You had an argument with your spouse or significant other; it was your birthday yesterday, and you made a serious departure from your nutrition regimen; you have a cold; your boss told you this morning that your paperwork was moving too slow; you're in the 10th week of a hurry-up, tight-deadline, 10-week project. Every day in your life is not the same.

Certain aspects of your fitness program, however, *are* the same, every time. Don't look at it as dreariness. Look at it as something dependable in an undependable world. Or as order amid chaos. Look at it as what a great musician, who performs to cheering crowds in concert halls around the world, does behind the scenes. Except that you've got it made compared to the great musician. Everything is turned around backwards in your favor. For every minute he's on stage, he has practiced scales for hours on end. For every week you're on stage, you spend just a few hours in the gym. You're practicing for *life.*

We're going to talk in this chapter about some of the basic elements and principles that make up a solid, safe, productive workout. We'll talk in terms of being in the gym, but you'll see that 90 percent of these pointers will apply if you're working out in your basement. We'll talk in terms of weight training, but you'll also see that 90 percent of what I say also applies to Dynabands and calisthenics and broomsticks and towels. These are the nuts and bolts of working out, and they are the same whether you are taking your first baby steps to fitness, or you've been pumping iron since gyms were invented.

PARTNERS

You can get fit, or sculpt your body to the best it can be, without ever once using a workout partner. But, man, is it easier—and safer—if you do the job two-by-two. I strongly recommend that everyone find a partner for his or her workout. A regular partner, of course, is the best.

Why is it best? For common-sense reasons.

Competition breeds success. This does *not* mean that when you enter the gym it's the bottom of the ninth, two out, bases loaded and you're the batter. It's not a *pressure* thing, it's a *motivational* thing. When that last set, or those ninth and 10th reps, require a little extra digging, it helps to have someone—even a friendly someone—on hand to see whether or not you do the work. (You're there for him or her, too, of course.) Don't forget that your partner is also in a "me vs. me" competition. He knows that it's not a question of whether you press 500 pounds, but how you stack up against yourself. When you make it through a routine with a 110-pound bar for the first time, you can *show off!* It works at every level—beginner or advanced. It's, "Look, Ma. No hands!" It's just plain psychological common sense.

Then there is what you might call the honesty factor. Not that I would accuse you of cheating. I certainly would never accuse anyone of cheating at golf, which is by reputation the most honorable of games. But how many strokes, on average, do you suppose we should add to all scorecards of golfers who play a round on their own?

Partners are a first-class safety factor. It's very much like swimming alone versus having a "buddy." You get cramps, or hit a sudden wall of fatigue, and somebody's there to bail you out. In weight training, it's called "getting stuck." People have been seriously injured, or killed, when they got stuck with hundreds of pounds of iron raised above their neck. I really don't recommend anyone *ever* working with heavy weights unless they have a partner. And common sense suggests that anyone undertaking heavy exertion of any kind should at least have someone else in sight in case they become distressed in any way. (Safety should be a concern in *any* kind of exercise. Cyclists, for example, should wear a helmet. If you don't, try this one on for size: *Football players* are smart enough to wear helmets.)

Finally, it's more *fun* to work out with a partner. It's like the difference between shooting hoops by yourself, or having a little game of one-on-one.

WARMUPS AND COOLDOWNS

A smart person doesn't hop into a $50,000 car on a cold February morning, start the engine and immediately see how quickly they can get from zero to 80 m.p.h. You don't do that to your body, either.

Warmups and cooldowns are a vital part of a routine, whether you are doing towel pulls in your dining room or pumping 300 pounds on a lat machine at the gym. Even if your entire routine consists of two songs' worth of hula hoop, you should begin and end with a few minutes of running in place, holding your arms out from your sides and wriggling them to loosen them up.

Get your heart rate up and get more blood in the muscles. Get your breathing up to speed. In the gym before a workout, do three to five minutes of a nice, even, slow-to-medium pace on an aerobics device—a stationary bike, a treadmill, or a stair machine.

Then do a few minutes of stretches. Muscles and tendons and ligaments can do an incredible amount of work. But do them a favor and help their elasticity—ease into it. It'll help prevent snapping and tearing when you get to the heavier part of your routine. There are a zillion stretches and many philosophies of stretching. A lot of it is idiosyncratic—meaning you find what's best for you. Make it a part of your self-education—from books and magazines, from personnel at your gym, from training partners, from self-experiment.

At the end of your workout, reverse the process. Do a couple minutes of stretches, then do 3 to 5 minutes of aerobic cooldown.

During your resistance-training workout itself, do a specific warmup for each exercise. In essence, do a super-light set (it doesn't count in your log or diary) that previews the movements for the muscle you are going to exercise. If it's a set of bench presses, for example, do a warmup set with just the bar, and no weights.

BREATHING

Key organs of the human body have all kinds of backup capacity that most people don't use. Being your best sometimes means tapping into this reserve. We use only a minuscule part of our brainpower, for instance. And the average person uses only about a quarter of his lung capacity. When you're working out, you want to get as close to 100 percent as possible.

Breathing properly is a basic, essential key to any exercise routine. Your body needs oxygen, and it's not going to come from anywhere else. Your body needs energy, and the fuel you put in your stomach is only part of it. This is the other part.

Breathe deeply though your nose. "Deeply" doesn't mean jerking your shoulders upward to draw a big breath. It means breathing from the *bottom* of your lungs, from the diaphragm. Expand your chest as far as you can. (As you "learn" to breathe, you're actually going to expand your rib cage and improve your posture.) While you're learning, you might even get a little light-headed—because you'll be high on oxygen.

There is an important rhythm to breathing while doing a routine. The best way to remember it is to *blow out on exertion*—in other words to exhale, strongly, during the hardest part of the movement. If you're doing bench presses, for example, blow out while you're raising the bar; inhale while bringing it back down. Practice the concept right now by doing some curling motions with your forearm. Force yourself to blow out while bringing your forearm up to your shoulder; inhale while lowering your arm. It might be just the opposite of your first inclination; but you'll feel the proper pattern, and get in tune with it, in just a couple of tries.

In the early days of your program, think about your breathing pattern constantly. Soon you'll be doing it right without thinking.

Remember, too, that proper breathing not only gets oxygen to your cells, it helps get wastes carried away. If you don't breathe efficiently, you're going to be much more sore the next day. That's why all those huffing and puffing aerobic dancers avoid post-workout pain.

BODY PARTS

Being fit gets you in touch with your body. Designing a workout program gets you in touch with your muscles in an almost clinical, analytical way. There are six major muscle groups to be worked, and every exercise is aimed at one or two of them. More advanced exercises are aimed at specific parts of one muscle. In the routines I've designed, beginners work on all six major groupings in each session. As you become more advanced, and the work becomes more intense, that number decreases. For example, in my own training I work on two body parts per session.

The major groupings are chest, triceps, legs, back, shoulders, biceps. There are subgroupings, of course, such as calves and stomach. The object of a good beginner's program is to train—in a plain, simple, fun fashion— the entire body in a symmetrical way.

Study. Ask questions. Resistance training, in all of its forms, has very specific goals for each movement. Know what it is that you are accomplishing, and you'll have more motivation to get it done.

REPS AND SETS

This is where you keep score. Except the goal isn't to "beat" the prescribed number of reps and sets. It's to do them exactly as programmed. As you progress, the program changes.

The next chapter includes some of the workouts I've designed and used with considerable success over the years for everyone from beginners to advanced lifters. You'll see that the guts of each workout look incredibly simple: so many sets of a certain exercise, so many repetitions per set. But those numbers are very important. The number of repetitions in a set of a particular resistance exercise, in fact, determines what it is that you are doing to your body.

Here are the basic principles of reps—keeping in mind that more reps, of course, are done with less weight; and that larger muscles can handle, and need, more sets.

Is strength all you want? Do you want to bulk up? Then pure, unadulterated anaerobic exercise—quick, maximum bursts of effort—is the ticket. The power-lifters, the grunters for whom how many pounds they can hoist into the air is everything, look at eight reps as a *long* set.

Is definition and endurance your goal? You want to get your musculature "cut" or "ripped"? Then you're looking at basic sets of about 15 reps.

For me, 10 is a magic number. A set of 10 reps builds strength and builds muscle, but it also builds definition. In any basic program, think of sets made up of 10 reps each. Muscles that need more work get more sets.

Ten reps is a number *infinitely* more important than the number of pounds you are lifting. Gauge it this way, no matter what movement you are making: The eighth, ninth and 10th reps should be difficult. (To the point where an 11th might not be possible, or only with utmost effort.) When you are fitting that formula, the work you are doing is right for that muscle—whether the weight on the bar says 50 or 300. Ten is a magic number, and might be the most important thing to remember from this entire chapter.

Never sacrifice style for weight. If your biorhythms are down, or if maybe you haven't been able to get as much sleep as you should, remove some pounds from the bar if that's what it takes to get to 10. On the other hand, if you do 10 reps and put the bar down when you could be doing five more—then you should have added weight a long time ago.

Ten reps will break down muscle and stimulate growth of new, larger, stronger tissue. Remember to blow out on the toughest part of every movement, oxidizing the blood with each thrust of energy.

The number of sets is largely determined by the size of the muscle. The smaller the muscle, the quicker it will become over-trained. That's why a program might call for six sets of a shoulder exercise, and 12 or 15 sets for a leg exercise.

Don't forget that every single principle of reps and sets applies to manual resistance training—Dynabands and towels and broomsticks. The magic number is still 10. And if you're a couch potato, you'll actually be getting enough resistance to build muscle.

REST

Two different kinds of rest are vital to any workout program: rest between sets, and rest between workouts. Beginners need more of both.

Taking no more than 30 to 60 seconds between sets keeps you from losing the "pump"—from losing oxygen-rich blood flow to the muscles you are working. Beginners will need all 60 seconds as a target rest period. If you're far enough out of shape, you'll not only be sucking wind, you'll hit your anaerobic threshold. You might experience some nausea, dizziness, headache, a cold sweat. If you lose your cookies, you won't be the first. Maybe not even the first of the day. It's very normal. It's your body saying: "Wait a minute!"

You have to start out by getting your mind in tune with the fact that this is, say, a 40-minute workout; that it's a lot more than just the first exercise. Then you have to push your body, but not kill it. Let me try to put all this in perspective by telling you what typically happens with personal training clients who come straight from 30 years at the office to their first day in a conditioning program. What I try to do—what all good personal trainers do—is try to work them to the max, short of hitting that wall. They come in all rambunctious. They're paying me by the hour. They want to get it on. But I fake them out a little, give them as much confidence as possible, keep them from feeling intimidated—but only give them *half* the workout. Next time, they get more.

Get the picture? *You* are the sculptor in every step of this conditioning process. You will constantly get in greater touch with your body. In the first workout or two, it might be more like your body slapping you in the face. You have to have patience with your body, listen to it, push it but don't insult it. You have to *wean* into fitness. You want to be back in the gym again and again for the rest of your life. Don't intimidate your body into refusing to bring you back.

I do "instinctive training." If I'm supposed to be doing five sets of one particular exercise, and if I lose "the pump" after four sets, I drop it. I move on. I've reached the plateau for that exercise. It takes *years* to be that in tune with your body. It's worth it in so many ways. Like when peer pressure or convenience tells you to pick up a double cheeseburger. A fit body tells you many things you can't hear just yet.

Rest between workouts is also crucial. A beginner will need 24 to 36 hours to recuperate. It takes me 12 hours—but again, it took me years to get to that point. Most beginners I put on a three-day-a-week program, two exercises per body part, two to three sets per exercise, 10 reps per set, 30 to 60 seconds between sets. That will build a foundation. There will be soreness in the first few rest days, but it will quickly diminish as you continue to work out.

SUPERSETS, TRI SETS, GIANT SETS

These exercises have a kind of Superman sound to them, but they are really just the opposite of power-lifting. They add aerobics and endurance conditioning to resistance training. They are very effective for athletes in endurance sports, who also want to add to their strength. I used supersetting, for example, to help condition a pro basketball player who was coming back from an achilles tendon injury.

Supersets are nothing more than two different exercises, one set each, done back to back without rest. I use supersets myself for aerobic conditioning. And in the final weeks before a bodybuilding competition I use tri sets (three exercises back to back with no rest) and giant sets (four or more) to add tremendous definition to the musculature I have built in months of workouts.

The intensity in supersetting is immense, but there's no reason to be wary. The most effective supersetting is done on the *same* body part—chest, for example—in two different exercises. You'll be dissecting the muscle, exercising it in separate places, using its reserve energy and bringing it to maximum exhaustion. That's the key.

Any workout should aim to get in and out of the gym quickly—building muscle without overtraining, or getting stale, or getting bored. Neither you nor your muscle will get bored with supersets. In fact, you'll "confuse" the muscle and fake out its "memory"—the reason your body becomes immune to a single exercise routine if you follow it too long.

A superset shocks the body, throws it a curveball. Doing two different exercises back to back with *no rest* moves the intensity from second gear to fifth gear. You'll be cross-training, doing aerobics and anaerobics simultaneously.

You use less weight and, once again, the magic number of 10. When you complete one superset, you take the usual rest period (30 to 40 seconds, because you'll be conditioned before you do supersets). That's a fast pace, and you'll probably be sucking wind. Your cardiovascular endurance will thank you for it.

Bodybuilders aren't building muscle with supersets and lighter weights, they're sculpturing—which is why it's a pre-contest routine. As a combined endurance/strength workout, it's dynamite for a triathlete, a downhill skier, a tennis player or a basketball player.

Because of supersetting's aerobics component, it's also the perfect exercise for someone who wants resistance training but also wants to lose some weight. A moderate-carb, protein-adequate, low-fat nutrition regimen and a gym regimen of supersets will make him or her one lean person.

SAFETY

Gyms can be dangerous places. So can cars. Defensive drivers who wear their seat belts shouldn't be afraid to drive to the grocery store. So it goes with gym training.

Some basic points:

- Make sure you are constantly bending your knees while doing any standing exercises. Your knees will act as a shock absorber. Otherwise your back will take the weight like throwing cement into a truck with no springs.

- Don't lock out on certain movements. For example, military shoulder presses, squats, leg presses.

- Wear a belt that's four inches wide. It'll also help protect your back. Anything wider than four inches will limit your range of motion.

- If you don't want calluses, wear a snug pair of gloves. If you wish, use a little chalk for a better grip.

- Wear loose clothing. You want good circulation and ventilation. Your arm can expand as much as an inch or inch and a half in the course of a workout, by the way.

- Wear sneakers or running shoes, with the laces well-tied. You want support and you don't want to trip.

- Wear gym socks to absorb sweat so you don't get bacterial infection.

- Always use a collar on a bar or adjustable dumbbell and fasten it tight to keep weights secure. That seems simple enough, but I've seen careless people splatter their face with a dumbbell.

- When you're walking around a gym don't lean against equipment unless you very consciously know exactly what the equipment is and what you are doing. Gym equipment has moveable parts. Some are chain-driven, for example. You could leave a finger in there if someone decided to lift while your hand was in the way.

- Keep a towel to wipe off your own sweat, or somebody else's, from a device or a bar you are about to grip or a bench you are about to lie on.

- Don't work beyond your comfort zone in hot and humid weather. "No pain no gain"—if you follow it out the window—is a fallacy. If something is painful while you're exercising, slow down or stop until the pain subsides. Overuse of muscles can cause damage or make you abandon your program.

DIARY

Whether it's a 49-cent spiral notebook or an executive logbook, this is one powerful tool. To my mind, it's absolutely essential for a successful program. You *are* going to make progress. But without a diary, you'll be at times like a ship passenger looking out at the ocean to see how far you've gone.

Use the diary to keep an accurate record of when you work out, what exercises you do, how many sets and reps, what poundage you use. Keep notes of what seems to be working and what doesn't. At the end of a session, if you think you're ready to make a change in a particular exercise next time, note it down so that you do. Write down questions you want to ask a trainer or instructor who isn't handy at the moment.

You might find it useful to combine a nutritional diary with your exercise diary. You should be keeping both. Some people find it easiest to put them in the same place; some find it more difficult.

Progress is all about goal-setting. After you've worked out a few months, and you hit a psychological down point (we all do), almost nothing will help you out as much as looking in your log. You'll see where you were. You'll remember why you're doing this. And you'll understand that, yes, you're getting there.

FLUIDS AND FUEL

Drinking fluids before, during and after a workout is important. So is the timing of your food intake. Be sure to refer back to Chapter 11 for details.

19

Five Levels, Five Programs —

Detailed Workouts for Various Levels of Fitness

Every body is different. Whether you are training at your home alone, at a gym with a partner, or with a personal trainer, you'll find ways of customizing any exercise regimen to your needs. In fact, you'll be changing your routine from time to time just to fight off that old enemy, boredom. So it's impossible to line up a set of exercises on the pages of a book and say: "Here; this is what you should do."

What we *can* do is take a look at five very different programs for five very different people. If you fit the profile of any of these people, you could pick up the routine and use it just as it's written. Very soon, however, you would begin to alter the routine, gradually, to match your progress, your current interests, any upcoming competitions or lifestyle changes, etc. Creativity in the gym is just as important as creativity in your nutritional regimen. You don't want to go stale and get off track.

MANUAL RESISTANCE ROUTINE

Remember, manual resistance is a great exercise tool for anyone from couch potato to football player to bodybuilder. This routine makes use of three pieces of equipment: a bath towel, a broomstick and a Dynaband. Keep in mind that Dynabands come in three different resistance strengths to match your physical condition.

This routine works out all the basic body parts and is perfect for a beginner—who should seriously consider working out with a partner, both for motivation and for fun. More advanced conditioners should never scoff at manual resistance training. It'll help keep you toned, and it means you never have an excuse for missing a workout, no matter where you are. Remember, an experienced gym rat can replicate almost any weight resistance exercise with a manual resistance equivalent.

CHEST	EXERCISE
3 sets of 10 reps	Flat flyes done on bench or floor, with Dynaband or with hand resistance

Lie back on the floor or on a bench, holding the Dynaband in each hand above the chest with a palms-in grip. Slowly lower Dynaband out and down until arms are parallel to the floor, maintaining a slight bend in the elbows. When pectorals are fully stretched, change direction and raise back up while tightening the chest muscles. Always take a deep breath as you move downward; blow out and constrict the muscle as you move up. That's one rep. (Without a Dynaband, have your partner provide hand resistance to both downward and upward movements.)

SHOULDERS	EXERCISE
3 sets of 10 reps	Seated military shoulder press, behind neck with broomstick (requires partner for resistance)

Sit down against back of chair to keep back straight and to provide support. Grasp broomstick with hands slightly beyond shoulder width. Begin with stick behind head and almost touching vertebra at base of neck. Push up. As you're thrusting up and blowing out, your partner provides resistance. When you get the broomstick three-quarters of the way to full extension, start bringing it back down. (Do not lock out elbows, or you could injure yourself.) Your partner, of course, must provide resistance in both upward and downward movements.

BACK	EXERCISE
3 sets of 10 reps	Towel pulls

BICEPS	EXERCISE
3 sets of 10 reps	Biceps curls, with towel or broomstick or Dynaband

For curls, stand upright, or sit, holding broomstick, towel or Dynaband in a shoulder-width grip with palms up. Your partner will have a close grip, palms down. Raise hands while keeping elbows locked to your sides so the only part of the arm you're using is from hand to elbow, with the elbow serving as pivot. Constrict the biceps as you raise broomstick or Dynaband or towel almost under your chin. Lower arm nice and slow—all the way until device touches thigh. That's one rep. Blow out coming up, the toughest part of the motion.

TRICEPS   EXERCISE
3 sets of 10 reps   Triceps pushdown, with towel or broomstick or Dynaband

Instead of palms facing you, as in curls, place your hands—and thumbs—over the towel or stick or Dynaband. Use a close grip, with your hands touching each other. Your partner uses a wide grip, outside your hands. (As you do triceps, he or she does biceps.) Keep your elbows tucked into your sides, as if a pin went through your body to keep them in place. As you move downward you do want to lock out, to squeeze and constrict the triceps. Do not take elbows away from sides as you come up.

LEGS   EXERCISE
3 sets of 10 reps   Side leg lifts, with Dynaband or hand resistance; leg extensions, with towel or hand resistance

For leg lifts, lie on side with Dynaband totally encircling both ankles. (Without a Dynaband, have partner supply resistance.) Lift leg in a "splits"-type movement, then turn on other side and repeat set with other leg. This is great for hips and buttocks.

To build the quadriceps (front of thighs), do leg extensions. Sit down on chair with resistance of hand or someone holding a towel over your ankles. Keeping the back part of your knee touching the end part of the chair, bring legs up together with toes pointed upward. Squeeze the quadriceps. And do lock out at the top, hesitating for a second while squeezing the muscle.

HAMSTRINGS   EXERCISE
3 sets of 10 reps   Resistance with hands, towel or Dynaband

Lying on your stomach, you move against resistance to the back part of the ankle as you raise the lower legs upward, using the knee as pivot point. Raise both legs together, from knee to ankle. Then move back down—again against resistance. This exercise strengthens lower back as well as hamstrings.

BEGINNER'S WEIGHT PROGRAM

This is one I designed for a corporate fitness program, but it's basically adaptable for any beginner. Remember, it's not about the amount of weight; it's about the reps and the magic number 10. Do *not* injure yourself by starting out with too much poundage. You can always add more until the ninth and 10 reps are difficult. That will be your benchmark for the time being.

All of my beginner's programs are designed for three days a week, Monday-Wednesday-Friday or Tuesday-Thursday-Saturday. Those two days off at the end of the cycle aren't just for scheduling convenience. They represent a proper cycle of rest.

This program is suitable for anyone who has never picked up a weight, or has been away from resistance training for a year or more. It will build a great foundation for moving on to the next plateau.

Warm up for five minutes on a stationary bike. Cool down after workout for five minutes on the stairs or a stair machine.

CHEST	EXERCISE
A: 2 sets of 10 reps	A: Inclined bench press with barbell
B: 2 sets of 10 reps	B: Flat dumbbell flye

For the bench press, use a 45-degree incline. Lie back and hold a weighted barbell above the chest at arm's length, gripping a little beyond shoulder width. Slowly lower the bar to the chest by bending the elbows. Lightly touch the bar against the upper chest, then press back upward until arms are straight. Pause and repeat. Blow out on exertion, going up.

For the flye, lie back on flat bench holding a dumbbell in each hand above the chest with a palms-in grip. Slowly lower the weights out and down until the arms are parallel to the floor, maintaining a slight bend in the arms to avoid hurting arms or shoulders. When the pectorals are fully stretched, change direction and raise the weights back up, tightening your chest muscles.

BACK	EXERCISE
A: 2 sets of 10 reps	A: Wide-grip barbell bent-over rows
B: 2 sets of 10 reps	B: Lat machine pulldown behind neck

For the bent-over rows, stand on the floor or on a raised platform to get more of a stretch. Bend forward, keeping knees slightly bent. (This will serve as a shock absorber.) Grasp weighted barbell with wide overhand grip and lift bar slightly while your back is parallel to the floor. Keeping the back flat, exhale and bend arms to lift the bar until it is near the stomach.

Inhale as you lower bar to starting position without letting the weight touch the floor. That's one rep.

For the pulldowns, sit at a lat pulldown machine gripping the long bar with a wide, open-handed grip. Place your thighs under the pads to hold the body down as you pull. Begin with arms straight over your head. Pull down by bending the elbows and squeezing the lat, stopping when the bar touches the back of the neck. Stretch the arms back out and repeat.

TRICEPS EXERCISE
A: 2 sets of 10 reps   A: Dumbbell kickbacks
B: 2 sets of 10 reps   B: Triceps dips

For the kickbacks, grasp a dumbbell you can handle easily with one arm. Assume a bent-over position on a bench or stool or chair. Place one foot 12 inches in front of the other, with your upper body parallel to the floor. Hold the dumbbell with an overhand grip, taking care to keep your upper body and elbow in line, with your forearm hanging straight down. That's the position.

The movement: While keeping your body still and upper arm tucked into your side, exhale and extend the arm (the only part of the arm that's moving is from elbow to wrist) to the rear until the arm is straight back. Inhale and return the dumbbell to the bottom position. After doing 10 reps, switch arms. This one will work the entire triceps.

For the dips, place two benches parallel and three to four feet apart. Support yourself on both benches—legs straight out and feet on one bench, hands behind hips on the other bench. Keeping the upper body erect, bend the elbows and lower your buttocks down near the floor. Use triceps to push back to straight-arm position. Inhale moving down; exhale moving up. Squeeze triceps at the top. For added resistance you can place a weighted dumbbell or a plate on your thighs. This is a simple exercise you can do at home using chairs or a bed. The closer your arms are behind you, the harder the effort on your triceps.

BICEPS EXERCISE
A: 2 sets of 10 reps   A: Standing barbell curls (medium grip)
B: 2 sets of 10 reps   B: Alternate dumbbell curls, seated

For the barbell curls, stand with feet at shoulder width, gripping bar at thigh level—with elbows nearly straight, palms facing upward and hands just outside the hips. Keeping the back straight, exhale and curl bar up to chest by bending elbows. Stop when biceps come fully tight, and do not let them relax by resting the bar against your chest. Lower bar while inhaling.

This simple, classic exercise is great for building big biceps.

For the alternate dumbbell curls, sit upright on a bench or chair holding a dumbbell in each hand with a palms-in grip. Keeping the right hand immobile, twist the left hand so palm faces you and lift the dumbbell by bending the elbow. Squeeze at the top so you are flexing the muscle. Pause and lower to original position. Repeat with opposite arm, and continue to alternate.

SHOULDERS	EXERCISE
A: 2 sets of 10 reps	A: Seated military shoulder press
B: 2 sets of 10 reps	B: Dumbbell side lateral

For the press, sit on a flat bench with barbell resting on shoulders and gripping bar beyond shoulder width with palms facing forward. Keep back straight and feet planted firmly on the floor. Exhale as you press the bar to arms' length in a controlled manner. Inhale and slowly return the bar to starting position.

For the lateral, stand with legs spread wide, knees slightly bent and back upright. Hold a dumbbell in each hand with palms facing the body. Breathing through your nose, inhale as you slowly raise dumbbells up and out to the sides, stopping when arms are at ear height. Hold for a count of three seconds, then slowly lower weights back to starting position. Keep thumbs pointed upward at all times. Beginners may lift to a point parallel to floor and try to go higher as they become stronger. In any case, never lift above your head in this exercise.

LEGS	EXERCISE
A: 2 sets of 10 reps	A: Leg extensions
B: 2 sets of 10 reps	B: Leg curls

Extensions will build the outer front thigh, the quadriceps. Sit at a leg extension machine with your insteps behind the roller pads and your hands gripping handles at the side of machine. Slowly straighten legs to lift the weights, keeping toes pointed up. Stop when knees are locked and quadriceps are flexed. Pause and lower, under control, to starting position without letting the weights come to rest. This exercise increases overall knee strength, boosts vertical jump and helps running speed. Be sure to adjust the leg extension seat so the back of the knee is snug against the front edge of seat. The bottom pad should be just above the ankle area but below the shin. Keeping your toes standing at attention makes sure that you work the entire quadriceps. Use a fluid, slow motion.

For the second exercise, lie on a leg hamstring curl machine with your heels beneath the roller pad and your chest flat on the bench pad, holding onto handles for support. Exhale and bend knees to lift pad as far as possible. Hold the flex position momentarily before inhaling and lowering to starting position. The kneecap should be just off the pad, or you'll hurt your knees. Keeping the heel tucked in isolates the muscle you're working. Make sure that it's a fully controlled, fluid motion.

STOMACH

2 giant sets, all to failure

NIELSEN'S TRI SET

A: Leg raises on stand
B: Crunches (legs on bench)
C: Sit-ups on board

Unlike all other muscles, the stomach area should be worked to failure instead of counting reps and resting between sets. As soon as you reach failure on one exercise, you move on to the next.

First, do leg raises on a legstand and work the stomach from the belly button down, attacking that little pouch area that a lot of people want to tone up. Because they work the lower abs best, knee-tuck leg raises should be done first in routine. Position yourself on a standing abdominal chair, supporting body weight on the forearms and hanging the straightened legs downward. Keeping your knees nearly straight, exhale and bend at the hips, lifting the legs out and up in front of you until they are parallel to the floor. Pause and inhale while returning to starting position. Immediately repeat, using a slow motion to work the abs better and ease strain off the lower back.

Next do crunches with your legs on a bench and your back firmly on the floor so your body lies in three nearly straight lines—torso on the floor, hips to knees straight upward, knees to feet on the bench and parallel to the floor. Position your butt very near the bench (or the bed or couch; this is an exercise you can easily do at home). Make relaxed fists and cross your hands on your chest to centralize your weight.

Your arms weigh at least three to five pounds, and you don't want to put them behind your head as in a traditional sit-up. To start, push your neck forward, then—from the middle of your back to the shoulders—raise your upper torso three to four inches and *squeeze* (simultaneously blowing out). That's the crunch. Kind of like half a sit-up, squeezing the muscles together. It's great for the stomach muscles from the belly button up. It's also "patient friendly" for people who have back problems.

For the sit-ups, never use a board slanted more than 45 degrees. This exercise works the entire stomach, but again focuses from the belly button upward. Again, centralize your weight by crossing your fists over your chest. Sitting on a slanted board, go down just halfway, inhaling. Blow out as you come up fully and extend your neck so you're actually squeezing stomach muscles. As you blow out, you constrict stomach muscles and put tension from your own weight on your abdominals. Do this to failure—till you get that burn in your stomach.

CALVES	EXERCISE
3 sets of 10	Seated calf raises

Sit on a calf-raising machine with your knees under the pads and the balls of your feet on the front platform. Lift weights by raising the toes. Unlock the holding bar. Begin with heels lowered so that the calves are stretched. Exhale and lift the weight by flexing the calves and lifting heels as high as possible. Squeeze momentarily, then lower to stretch position while inhaling. Do three sets: first with feet straight second with toes and feet facing inward, third with feet facing outward. This develops the full calf muscle.

INTERMEDIATE WEIGHT PROGRAM
A person undertaking this program probably has been involved in weight training for at least a year. He or she already has built enough endurance to train four days a week instead of three—and will be familiar with most exercise terminology. (In any case, I won't define or explain movements we've already discussed.)

By going to a four-day-a-week program, he or she is taking a serious step. Following this routine will allow you to be the sculptor, to customize your body—for size, strength, toning, speed, or for competition in any sport.

The program is designed for rest days on Wednesday, Saturday and Sunday. Day One of the routine (chest, triceps and legs) is done on Monday and Thursday. Day Two (back, shoulders and biceps) is done on Tuesday and Friday.

Stretch and do at least five minutes on stairs, bike or treadmill for warm-up.

DAY ONE
CHEST:		
	A: Incline bench press with barbell	5 sets, 10 reps
	B: Incline dumbbell flyes	3 sets, 10 reps
	C: Flat bench press with barbell	5 sets, 10 reps
	D: Flat dumbbell flyes	3 sets, 10 reps

TRICEPS:	A: Over-the-head one-arm dumbbell triceps extensions	2 sets, 10 reps
	B: French press, lying down or on bench with close grip	3 sets, 10 reps
	C: Pushdowns on lat machine	3 sets, 10 reps

For the one-arm dumbbell triceps extensions, stand upright with your left hand on hip while holding a dumbbell above the head in the right hand. Begin with upper arm tucked into the ear, elbow bent so the weight is behind the head. Without moving the upper arm, exhale; then straighten the elbow until the weight is above you and triceps is flexed. Inhale while lowering back down behind the head, bending the arm only from the elbow to the wrist and extending the triceps. Your biceps remains tucked into the side of your head. Complete a set, then alternate with the other arm.

For the French press, lie down on a flat bench and grasp the barbell with a close grip, palms away from your body. Take the bar off the rack and hold it over your chest with arms fully extended. Your elbows are going to stay stationary and tucked, while your forearms lower the bar to forehead level. Inhale as you are coming down, blow out and extend the triceps as you go back up. In truth, this is a tough movement—and excellent triceps developer—in both downward and upward motions.

LEGS:	A: Squats	5 sets, 10 reps
	B: Leg extensions	4 sets, 10 reps
	C: Leg press	5 sets, 10 reps
	D: Leg curls	4 sets, 10 reps

For squats, hold the weighted barbell on your shoulders and assume a shoulder-width stance. Standing with your heels on a two-by-four will provide better leverage and put more emphasis on the quadriceps. Hold the bar beyond shoulder width, with palms over the bar, and keep the head up and back straight. Inhale deeply and bend your knees until your thighs are parallel to the floor. Do *not* take a full bend; it could hurt your knees. To gauge how deep you are squatting, put a bench behind you and let your buttocks brush the bench lightly. Change directions without bouncing. Exhale while pushing with legs back up to starting position. Don't lock out; keep the legs slightly bent.

For the leg press, sit at a 45-degree leg press machine with your back flat against the pad and feet at a shoulder-width stance on a movement platform. Push out until legs are straight, then turn the safety pin to release the free movement. Inhale and slowly bend legs until thighs approach chest at the bottom position. Exhale while pushing back up to starting position, but don't lock knees out. Do not lower weight too fast.

STOMACH: A: Seated leg kicks   3 giants sets, all to failure
B: Standing leg raises
C: Sit-ups on slant board

   For the leg kicks, sit on edge of bench with legs hanging off the end and hands grasping the bench behind the buttocks to support the body. Begin with legs lifted and slightly bent. Without moving the upper body, pull legs into your chest by bending at hips and knees. Concentrate on lower abdominal muscles, holding flex position for a moment and then slowly extending to start position before repeating. Do in a fluid motion until failure. Blow out as your knees are coming in to chest—that's when you constrict the lower abs.

DAY TWO
BACK: A: Lat machine, wide grip   2 sets front, 10 reps
2 sets rear, 10 reps
B: Lower cable rows to stomach 3 sets, 10 reps
C: Bent-over rows, wide grip   4 sets, 10 reps

   For lower cable rows, sit at a row station placing feet on pads and bending knees a bit. Grasp the close-grip handle with palms facing inward. Bend forward at the waist to stretch the lat and assume starting position. Pull the handle into the stomach area, simultaneously sitting upright without arching your back. Pause and stretch forward by bending your back once more before repeating. It's much like a rowing motion—you're sitting down, you're grabbing the handle, your knees are slightly bent on the pad. Your hands are going out and extending and bending from your hip area so your back is being pulled forward, then you're coming back and sitting up straight at attention. Bring the handles down to your belly button, then really flare and flex your back. Repeat.

SHOULDERS: A: Seated military barbell press   3 sets, 10 reps
B: Side dumbbell laterals   3 sets, 10 reps
C: Barbell or dumbbell shoulder shrugs 3 sets, 10 reps
D: Upright rows with barbell   3 sets, 10 reps

   Shrugs are just what the name suggests—trying to get your shoulders up to your ears without bending your arms at all. With dumbbells, you stand up with the weights at the sides of your body. Squeeze your shoulders up and down. The more advanced can rotate during the motion. If you're using a barbell, hold it forward against your thighs. You can get a better range of motion with dumbbells.

For upright barbell rows, stand upright with knees slightly bent. Hold the bar with overhand grip just inside the shoulders. Begin with arms straight, then lift weight upward by bending elbows while keeping the bar close to the body until it touches under chin. Pause and lower.

BICEPS: A: Biceps machine or preacher bench with barbell
                                                2 sets close, 10 reps
                                                2 sets wide, 10 reps
             B: Seated alternate dumbbell curls   3 sets, 10 reps
             C: Standing heavy curls with barbell   3 sets, 10 reps

With biceps machine, grab the bar (a close grip works the peak part of arm; a wide grip works inner part of biceps) and lean against the machine with armpits totally wedged against the pads and arms over the pads. Put *all* weight of chest against the pad so you can't cheat and use your back. Press elbows into pads, with arms fully extended down and grabbing onto the bar with underhand grip so fingers are facing you. Keep the elbows and back of triceps against the pad at all times. Keeping arms straight, come up with the bar underneath the chin. Squeeze and constrict. Come back down just three-quarters of your range of movement; if you come down all the way you could hyperextend the muscle. Exhale coming up; inhale as you're going down. What you're doing here is absolutely isolating the biceps and working it fully. (Do the same exercise with a bar on a preacher bench at a 45-degree decline. Don't swing your arms. Use a nice, fluid, slow motion. Constrict the muscle as you move up.)

CALVES: A: Standing calf raises   3 supersets, 10 reps
             B: Seated calf raises

Use a standing calf raise machine after adjusting upper pads so weights are lifted when you stand upright on a floor platform. Place your hands on the upper handles and begin with knees straight and heels lowered to get a full stretch. Without bending the knees, exhale and flex the calf until you are standing tiptoe. Hold momentarily before inhaling as you lower back to stretch your calf in the starting position. Use moderately heavy weight. For best unrestricted movement, do this one in bare feet.

ADVANCED WEIGHT PROGRAM

This individual has a foundation of at least two years' worth of weight training. Putting the proper rest interval into the program means that he or she will have to check the calendar to see which days are gym days. That's because it's a three-days-on, one-day-off, three-days-on, two-days-off regimen.

Note that at this plateau, you are down to two body parts per workout—each more thoroughly and intensively, allowing you to concentrate on your weak areas.

By now, you don't have to be reminded that you need to warm up (five minutes on bike) and cool down (five minutes on stairs).

DAY ONE

CHEST: 4 supersets, 10 reps each:
Incline bench press
Incline dumbbell flyes
4 supersets, 10 reps each:
Flat bench press to neck
Flat dumbbell flyes
2 sets of 10 reps each:
Decline dumbbell press, turn wrists in
at top position

SHOULDERS: Seated military press on machine or with barbell
3 sets, 10 reps:
Upright rows, barbell (narrow grip)
3 sets, 10 reps; vary position of grip after every set
Alternate dumbbell front and side laterals
2 supersets of 10 reps
Rear deltoid machine or bent-over rear side laterals
2 supersets of 10 reps
Barbell or dumbbell shrugs

CALVES: Seated and standing calf raises
4 supersets: in, out, straight; use different foot
positions

DAY TWO
BACK: Wide-grip chin-ups
                        4 sets, 10 reps
                   Wide-grip bent-over rows with barbell
                        4 sets of 10 reps
                   Lat machine, wide grip
                        3 sets in front, 3 in back
                   Lower cable rows
                        4 sets, 10 reps
                   Dumbbell alternate rows
                        2 sets, 10 reps

TRICEPS: 4 supersets of 10 reps:
                        Close-grip lat machine pushdowns
                        Dumbbell overhead triceps extensions (elbows
                        tucked into head)
                   3 supersets of 10 reps:
                        Seated triceps machine;
                        Reverse close-grip pushdowns
                   2 sets, 10 reps:
                        Alternate cable kickbacks

DAY THREE
BICEPS: 4 supersets; 2 close, 2 wide:
                        Cable curls with bar
                        Biceps machine or preacher bench
                   3 sets, 10 reps:
                        Seated alternate dumbbell curls
                   2 sets, 10 reps:
                        Concentrated curls

LEGS: Leg extensions, Smith machine   5 supersets, 10 reps each
                   3/4 squats
                   Leg press, leg curls   4 supersets, 10 reps each
                   Sissy squats   2 sets to failure

STOMACH: Sit-ups on slat board   3 giant sets, all till
                   Ab crunch on bench   failure
                   Standing leg-raisers
                   Sidebends on hyperextension

NIELSEN'S JUNIOR FITNESS ACADEMY

After all that advanced stuff, I want to include this simple little program. Fitness for kids is vitally important, no matter what activities we use to achieve it. Not all youngsters will take to the gym. But some will love it, and make it a lifetime program. Here's a basic workout for kids aged 6 and up.

Warm-up is 3 - 5 minutes on bike. Cool-down is 5 minutes on stairs.

A: Leg extensions	2 sets of 10 reps
B: Triceps pushdowns	2 sets of 10 reps
C: Seated alternate dumbbell curls (for biceps)	2 sets of 10 reps
D: Shoulder side lateral	2 sets of 10 reps
E: Wide-grip lat machine pulldowns	2 sets of 10 reps

When I hand kids a printed workout, the notes at the bottom remind them that workouts will:

1. Build discipline
2. Help correct poor posture
3. Build strength
4. Build confidence and self-esteem
5. Help fight obesity
6. Help control high cholesterol
7. Exercise the most important muscle: the heart.

20

Going All the Way

You're right. I'm an extremist.

As a pro bodybuilder, I've taken my own conditioning to the top one-tenth of 1 percent. As a nutrition counselor who walks what he talks, my daily menus look incredibly spartan compared with what everybody else on the block eats. As a human being, it actually *pains* me to see good people—successful people, smart people, educated people, kind people, thoughtful people—being dragged down by not taking care of their bodies.

Why am I in so deep? Why do I push so far? And what's the deal with that large number of people who go into the gym to lose a little flab, or to tone up a bit, or to regain some self-confidence—and wind up pushing farther than *they* ever imagined? What's with all these extremists?

The answers are at the core of my message. Understanding what drives us extremists will help you comprehend the gifts of fitness—no matter what path you choose to achieve it and whether or not you ever get within a mile of advanced weight training.

We're not talking muscleheads and gym rats—people for whom the gym is a pool hall, a place to hang out with their obsession. They do exist. Instead of being evenly yoked, they live only to pump iron.

We're talking accountants and broadcasters and business owners and housewives, people who live busy and fulfilling lives. Ninety-five percent of the time they never see a barbell. But for a half-dozen hours spread through each week, they are hard-core extremists, intensely devoted to a training regimen. They aren't just dabbling at the gym. They've moved upward from plateau to plateau to plateau without looking back. In most cases, no one is more surprised than themselves.

I rely on them to help explain what I'm about. I have to, because when I meet people outside the gym—in business, socially, or in speechmaking—there's an almost invariable pattern. First, they want to see if I can walk and chew gum at the same time. Then they want to see if I can carry on an intelligent conversation. Then, when I pass those tests, they come around a little bit. After all, *everybody* wants to be healthy. "You make a lot of sense, Peter," they'll say. "But why do you carry it *so far?* Who needs all those muscles?"

Let me get at it by telling you about the 25 percent. I can't exactly explain why, but about a quarter of my personal training clients wind up doing things that they never dreamed they'd do the day they walked in the door. I don't mean how many pounds of weight they lift, or whether some contest judges say they have the most symmetrical body on a stage. I mean in terms of a radically new attitude toward life.

Most come to me to lose a few pounds, or to firm up a bit, or because they're just tired of waking up tired. Almost everybody who lasts more than a few weeks benefits. They get into a program, they build a training foundation. All the physical things that happen—from metabolism to muscle tone—breed confidence and general well-being. For most people, that's plenty. But for this very large minority, this 25 percent, it's like they swallowed rocket fuel. Whooooosh! Look out, world.

Part of it is this: The *real* competition in the gym is with yourself. That is the toughest, most rewarding, most meaningful competition in all of sport. You can set a world record every day. If you start out doing 10 reps with 50 pounds, then the day you do 10 reps with 55 pounds breaks the world record by 10 percent. If 10 minutes on the treadmill leaves you sucking wind, then the day you do 15 minutes you have *destroyed* the world record. It's the only reasonable way to look at it. Put two sprinters up against each other, or two racehorses, or two football teams. One of them might win without doing his best. It happens every day. The *only* way you can *ever* beat yourself is by doing your best.

And then this marvelous thing happens. *Me vs. me* becomes fun. Fun the way that rewarding, hard work is fun. Me vs. me becomes satisfying, the way real food is satisfying and candy isn't. And your best keeps getting better. On to the next plateau.

I couldn't list all the triggers that get pulled and send people into the gym for the first time. Some go because their spouse left them. Or because they figured out that they're losing money because their boss doesn't like fat people. Or because their rear-end is too big and their self-esteem is too small. Or because they've just realized that an idle body goes straight downhill with age. Or because they're fighting Crohn's disease and are absolutely infatuated with the idea of being alive inside a healthy body instead of being trapped in a crumbling prison. A million reasons, some of them serious and some of them trivial, make people take that first step through the door. Nobody, unless they're delirious, has those higher plateaus in mind on that first day.

When it starts happening, when your best keeps getting better, you finally look around one day and say: "What the hey; I think I *will* be the best that I can be." It spills out all over the place. In your personal life and your business life. You are the world champion in me vs. me. A lot of self-doubts go down that shower drain every day you work out. Who needs arrogance? Energy will suffice; and you have a surplus.

It's that energized, confident atmosphere that ignites the rocket fuel for the 25 percent. Stand back, because liftoff is going to be spectacular. And not very predictable.

Take my friend in Brooklyn. He was 60 pounds overweight. He regarded bodybuilding as a modeling show from Mars. It was the last thing he ever expected to get involved in. And when he came to me for PT, it was the last thing *I* ever expected him to be involved in. He built a foundation. He committed himself to a program. He shed the fat. He said: "Hey, this is fun, this is rewarding." And he took himself to the next plateau. Then—in the kind of blast-off behavior that no longer blows my mind—he decided to enter a bodybuilding competition. Not that he had changed his mind about bodybuilding contests. He just wanted to prove something to himself. And he got up on stage and won his class.

Or take the woman client who came to me many pounds overweight. She was well-motivated and took to training like a bird takes to flight. She was disciplined and goal-oriented. But could I tell early on that she would be one of the 25 percent whose horizons and viewpoint would open up— BOOM—like the curtain on a play? No way. Until one day she revealed to me a new goal—not as a joke, not as a delusion, but as a calmly confident new goal. "I think I'd like," she said, "to pose for *Playboy*." At this writing, she hasn't. But she *could*. The fact that training made her physically qualified to pose as a model or a *Playboy* subject isn't half as interesting as the fact that it made her want to do something so audacious. We're talking major change in ways a lot more important than a muscle here and there.

Do people make choices and chart paths differently when they're in top shape than when they're badly out of shape? Absolutely. Fitness and its relationship to mental attitude is potent and complex. There is no question that fit people see things differently and react differently. Making your best better physically can totally rearrange the way you interact in your daily life. I've seen it turn self-second-guessers into straight-ahead doers. When someone takes the extra step, becomes one of that 25 percent, the results sometimes approach rebirth.

So I'm an extremist. I came at weight training, like most people off the street, in terms of turning a negative into a positive. I've told you more in this book about the specifics that led me to the gym than I've ever told anyone. Really. Some of my best friends are going to be amazed.

But these are things you have to understand if this book is going to accomplish any of the things I want it to accomplish. There are plenty of books and magazines, some of them very bad and some of them very good, that run cover to cover with detailed exercise routines. You can buy them at the corner drugstore. I had stacks of them down in my grandmother's basement. But they're sterile. They don't tell the story. My own routines and programs are first class. They're well thought out, based on 25 years of top experience, and they work. But no program is worth a penny unless you understand *why you should be working out*. Why you might become an extremist. Why you'll benefit even if you climb only half of the weight-training plateaus—or even if you just advance from couch potato to nutrition-conscious bicyclist.

I like to think the main reason I'm not a musclehead is I really believe that me vs. me is the competition that counts. I really do see world champions all over the place when I look around my gym. The body I live in is the result of the *Peter Nielsen Me vs. Me Competition*. Whether I ever win another trophy, or whether I ever did win a trophy, is not half as important as the fact that I am world champion of my own body. Nobody else can win that title. And I can't take away anybody else's.

I certainly can't win Chuck Robertson's title. Chuck is the *champion* extremist. He is in the top 1 percent of the 25 percent who decide to be the very best that they can be. My Crohn's problem looks like a head cold when you stack it up next to his spinal muscular atrophy (the Kennedy form, in medical terminology), a close cousin to Lou Gehrig's disease.

The traditional approach says a person with this disease shouldn't exercise. That tears down muscle—which is exactly what the disease is doing in its creeping, progressive march against the victim's body. But Chuck decided that instead of just putting his adversity in a closet and fading away, he would take charge and put it in front of him on a daily basis. He decided to learn all he could about nutrition and exercise. And he came to the gym to try to hold the disease in remission. We worked together, with his doctor's approval, on a fitness program.

In four to five months, Chuck lost about 30 pounds of *fat*. He began to feel better than he had in many years. And when he lifted that arm and flexed, there it was: nothing that's going to win any hardware or wind up on the cover of a muscle mag, but an honest-to-God toned biceps. Nobody has to ask Chuck why *he* pushed so far.

I later met with one of the country's top specialists in diseases of muscular atrophy to go over the documentation of Chuck's physical therapy. It may be that we broke some new ground. If so, it'll fit a pattern of modern medical knowledge that is ironic: In a nation turned couch potatoes, health care professionals more and more are prescribing exercise for patients who used to be sent to bed for days or weeks. Everybody by now either has experienced, or has seen a family member experience, the new regimen of getting up and strolling the hospital corridor within hours after surgery. Exercise is a wondrous thing.

Another businessman, only in his 40s, came to me for physical therapy after two strokes. He was almost to the point of needing a wheelchair and had lost much of his will to live. The doctors sent over his reports, let me know his limitations, and OK'd a more aggressive approach. I designed a dumbbell and machine workout program for him and he went into the *me vs. me* competition. He went from a walker to a cane. Because of the passion in that internalized competition, and the strength it brought to his body, he is now living a much more normal life. He is stone intent on being the best he can be. And his best has gotten much better. Another extremist.

I don't *need* all those muscles, not the way Chuck needs the ones he's working on. But the only real difference between us is that I was blessed with body tissue that allows my best effort to produce musculature. I thank God every day for that, and for the opportunity to work with people like Chuck.

Yeah, I enjoy strutting my stuff in a bodybuilding competition. I *love* speaking to an audience that wants to know whether I can walk and chew gum at the same time. I thrive on the fencing matches that we call "business." Confidence, after all, is borderline cockiness. The fitter I am, the more it's there. That's true, I am convinced, of anybody.

What I enjoy most is getting that message through to other people. That's probably my ultimate reason for being an extremist: It helps get the message across.

Some of the people who hear it become extremists, too, and do audacious things. Fun and flippant things. Profound and moving things. Like deciding to pose for *Playboy*. Or making a stricken body take strides it isn't supposed to take.

2 1

Fighting a Flabby Future

Here's a conversation my Brooklyn childhood friends and I never had after a spirited session of street hockey:

"Hey man! Are we gettin' our aerobics today, or what?"

"Yeah, man! Like, my heart's been at its ideal rate for an hour!"

"Yuh know, my basal metabolism rate is gonna be outta sight tonight."

It all would have been true, though. Street hockey was spontaneous, and we were having fun, but we were fitness freaks and didn't know it. We probably talked and yelled for a year without saying the word "fitness."

Video games hadn't been invented yet. Baseball was something kids played, not something that was on six TV channels seven nights a week. We weren't active because we were smart. We were active because *life* was active. Playing stickball and street hockey was like breathing.

In grade school, we went to Phys. Ed. classes *every day*, for 45 minutes. We had to. Today, in school district after school district, elementary physical education gets zero priority. In district after district, not even a weekly exercise session is required of all those high school kids who spend their lunch hours mainlining fat at the fast-food joints. Billions of dollars spent on education, and not five cents' worth of intelligence about the human body trickles down to the students.

What in the world is going on here? We've got a major crime in progress and nobody's stopping it. It looks to me—as I think it would to anybody who analyzed the scene with an open mind—like we're breeding a generation of computer-literate cardiac cases. We spend double-digit percentages of our national wealth now on health care. That's with millions of Americans still alive who grew up active and spent their lives working with their hands. What do you suppose the bill is going to be when everybody who grew up with a joystick in one hand and a cheeseburger in the other hits middle age? Parents and schools and every institution that has anything to do with our kids' well-being are going to have to answer some serious questions.

The days are long past when you could feed kids and let them run out the door to play, knowing the one thing they wouldn't be lacking when they came back was exercise. The more likely scenario now is slipping the kid a few bucks to buy his own grease and sugar, after which he or she plays computer games or watches music videos. And just when this huge fitness vacuum shows up among our youngsters, the schools practically walk away from the fitness business. Amazing.

There are laws, and proposed laws, around the country making it illegal for an owner to let a dog ride in the back of a pickup truck. People *argue* about these laws. The debate gets ink in the newspapers. Somebody gets *that* worked up about the health and safety of dogs, and I don't hear any outcry about the horror show that is our own kids' fitness! You tell me: If it's a $50 fine for letting your dog ride in the back of a truck, why isn't it a $5,000 fine for steering your 12-year-old child into a life of obesity, inactivity and future cardiac problems? Where are the priorities?

When the first baby-boomers started to hit middle age, we saw a mini-boom in exercise. You see a lot of affluent boomers at the health clubs, buying diet pills and workout videos, jogging and spinning. That's nice (except for the diet pills). But I haven't seen any statistics suggesting that the boomers are passing this newfound interest in fitness on to their kids. I know it's tougher these days to pass *any* kind of values on to youngsters. But we have to try harder. And we have to make fitness a whole lot bigger piece of the values picture for kids.

A young person probably will survive the wildest, trendiest music, the goofiest hairstyles, even the body piercing. He'll probably survive all the rites of passage. He'll probably get around the drug culture. Statistically, it looks like he stands a chance against the AIDS epidemic. Somewhere down the line, he'll get past all the booby traps and be a normal, functioning, productive adult. But he has to do all that, and then live the next 60 years or so *in the same body.* All of those scary things that your child must dodge or endure are real enough, but the fact is this: He's likely to have more sustained grief in his life because of his physical condition than because of all the rest of those obstacles put together.

Nobody has measured that, or written that, as far as I know. But think about it. There's a *long* road ahead after, say, age 21. More than two-thirds of the average American lifespan. Do you want your child running down that road on two cylinders half the time, and spending the other half the time in the repair shop? Of all the things you could pass on to your kids, shouldn't a passion for fitness be high on the list? Do you want your offspring *believing* that "life sucks, and then you die"? Nothing you hear on the street bugs me as much as that one. I can't prove it, but I *know* it's an attitude you almost never hear from somebody who takes fitness seriously. It makes sense if you have to drag your body out of bed and through the day. If you have energy to spare, and the positive force that comes with it, then it's a crock.

So how does a parent get the message across?

First, by not giving the opposite message. If a parent's own nutritional and exercise life is a disaster zone, then he or she is sending a loud and clear signal of the worst kind. Like everything else in parenting, suddenly you're not doing things just for yourself—you're doing them for those little people in the house who are all eyes and ears. You can't do anything about the million-dollar jock peddling junk food on TV, but you can do plenty about the mother and father peddling junk food in the living room. And you can keep your own role-model face from staring at the TV set for five hours a day.

Second, the good news is that the active state of mind is contagious among people living in close quarters. A lot of what passes for heredity is nothing but "inherited" *habits.* "Like father, like son" doesn't have much to do with genes. There are no "born tennis players," but there are thousands of them who were born to tennis-playing families.

Third, more good news is that fitness can be a catalyst for a lot of other things you want to achieve as a parent. You hear a lot about "family values" these days. I'm not sure what that is. Your family's values might not be exactly the same as mine. But for sure, it all starts with the family being together. If you don't count TV watching (which I don't), family togetherness has become a rare event. Well, being active and being fit can make togetherness happen. A parent and a teen might have a tough time finding music they want to listen to together, but jogging, as one active example, is a different story. An entire family can hike together, or canoe together. Everybody in the canoe is getting fit; but they're also *talking,* sharing, understanding.

Grandparents need a footnote, by the way. Here's Grandpa, who spent 30 years unloading trucks and now spends two hours a day bending over and weeding his garden. For his age, he's probably more fit than 98 percent of the kids in America. He loves his grandchildren. So what does he do for the 8-year-old? He keeps him supplied with every video game known to man. The old smother-'em-with-love problem has its special twists these days. Parents have to let the older generation know what's up. Put the video away, and let the kids go help Grandpa plant his zucchini.

Schools live in close quarters with kids for more hours a week than parents do. And somewhere along the line our schools have lost sight of producing a sound mind in a sound body. Educators are absolutely right when they throw a lot of blame for their failures back at parents. Parents who don't read generally have kids who don't read. Parents who are couch potatoes have kids who are couch potatoes. But the last time I looked, schools were still trying to teach kids to read. Meanwhile, many schools are doing no job, or at best a poor job, of teaching kids to be fit.

How can a school district not have a physical education requirement? It's insane. We're always looking to other countries for a rallying cry. If Germany or Japan teaches more math than we do, then it's a national disgrace for us. How about Phys. Ed? All these countries that put more into their kids' brains put more exercise into their kids' bodies, too. Why aren't we upset about that? Why do we even need to look overseas? Study after study tells us what we already know: Our kids are inactive, and their bodies are paying the price. The real bill is going to come due in about 20 years. It seems obvious to me that we have to make Phys. Ed. a mandatory part of the curriculum in all of our schools.

That's just for starters. Then there's the matter of *what kind* of Phys. Ed. classes we offer. Here are three Phys. Ed. teachers I've run into. They're real people, but they're also types. You'll find them—and variations—in school gyms all around the country:

Teacher A is a football coach, or an ex-football coach. He wants to teach 12- or 13-year-old kids that gang calisthenics are the way to stay fit. All together now, hup, two, three, four. Teacher B is a power lifter. He thinks the way to go is to teach kids to do short sets and add weight. For him, strength is where it's at. Teacher C is a gymnast. She opposes resistance training and is really into stretching. She obviously teaches quite a different way. It's as if we had some schools teaching that the Earth is flat, some that the Earth is round, and some that it's shaped like a kiwi.

We need to get everybody on the same page and frequency. You can't have kids from one school coming home and trying to bench press as much weight as they can, and kids from another school thinking that fitness means military push-ups. We need some shared standards and some shared goals. And then maybe—since it seems like everything in education sinks or swims on a national wave—Phys. Ed. departments would have the clout at budget time to get equipment and salaries that are needed for a good program.

When I talk to school assemblies—which I do several times a year—I give a three-part message: nutrition, exercise and motivation. I tell them they may not be the *best* at throwing a baseball or running a mile, but by being active they can be *the best they can be*. I tell them that pigging out on junk food isn't half as pleasurable as feeling good and looking good because you eat right. Ninety-nine percent of the kids love it. Ninety-nine percent of the teachers love it. But nobody adds a Phys. Ed. requirement the next day. What happens the next day is that the PTA or the Band Boosters need to raise money. And how do they do it? By having all the moms send in layer cakes and peanut butter cookies to sell to the kids. Let's get serious!

Privately, many Phys. Ed. teachers tell me they just can't fight the bureaucracy. That there's no money for a program. That Phys. Ed. always has been and always will be the least glamorous and least respected job in the schoolhouse. That qualifications for leading a couple of hundred kids toward lifetime fitness are not always the qualifications that land the job.

These are big-time hurdles, and there are lots of dedicated teachers out there trying to jump them. They need some support from parents. That doesn't mean the Letter Club raising money so a few football players can wear NFL-type uniforms. It means a community's taxpayers saying: "We want our kids, all of them, to graduate with a sound mind in a sound body. We want our kids, after maybe $100,000 worth of education, to know nutritional poison as well as they know the multiplication tables. We want our kids to graduate with the cardiovascular health of an 18-year-old, not a 40-year-old. We want our kids to be thinking about fitness now, not after their first coronary."

That would be my dream—one big, squeaky wheel demanding and getting the grease it deserves.

Meanwhile, as a parent, do what you can on the homefront. Remember that togetherness and fitness go together like a bat and ball. If you really want to try something cool, radical and audacious, suggest to your teenage son or daughter that you launch a conditioning program together. Remember manual resistance-towels, broomsticks and Dynabands? *Great* conditioning for a teenager, as well as for you. And both of you need a training partner, so there you go.

If the idea of conditioning with Mom or Dad is just *too* far out for either child or parent, encourage your youngster to find another partner, to start a conditioning diary and go at it. An amazing thing: I've seen parents encourage their kids to take piano or art lessons or to go to the museum or to build model airplanes, but I don't even need all the fingers on one hand to count the times I've seen a parent encourage a kid to work out! In fact, I've seen parents discourage it. "It'll stunt growth," they say. Or: "Growing bodies can't handle it."

That's pure nonsense. True, young people shouldn't be doing any weight resistance training above their head before the age of about 17. That leaves 99.9 percent of the conditioning arena open to teenagers. And there are a zillion ways to get children into an active, conditioning state of mind between the ages of 6 and 13, when they are most impressionable and likely to form lifelong habits. A few *pre-school* programs have designed activities around the idea of just getting together—including parents in the picture—and being active. Some specific resistance training can be appropriate as young as 6 or 7. Some sections of the country have junior fitness academies with formal workout programs.

You have no reason to fear harming a young child by encouraging him or her to try towel pulls, push-ups, sit-ups, running in place, riding a bike or playing soccer. Activity is the main thing, and aerobic activity will strengthen the youngster's heart, improve metabolism and encourage a good night's sleep. You want one of the really great workouts? Try a brisk session of jumping rope. And then remember that when you encourage your child to do it, there's a whole lot more going on than "going out to play."

Organized physical activity—whether it's a structured workout or playing on a soccer team—brings a dimension of mental development, discipline and a sense of responsibility. A child who is learning to take care of himself, to be more in tune with his or her body, is more likely to take care of and respect others. That comes from learning to respect himself, which is one of the great contributions of sports.

You can roll your eyes and say that sports are hideously overemphasized in this country, and you know something? I'd agree with you 100 percent. Except that "sports" is the wrong word in that sentence. *Watching* sports events and glamorizing the superstars is hideously overemphasized in this country. Some of the roundest couch potatoes in the universe think they're into sports. They're not. They're into watching. That's a different ballgame. Guzzling beer, holding a finger in the air and screaming: "We're number one!" is not sports. Being into sports, for my money, means you play a team game, or you work out, or you run. The geeks who guzzle beer and watch 50 games a week seldom do any of those things. And they give sports a bad name.

Maybe that's why soccer intrigues me as a fitness sport for kids, even though I never played the game. Hundreds of thousands of youngsters across the country play this sport—even though not one parent in 100 ever played it, and even though you need a satellite dish and a foreign language translator to pick it up on your TV. It requires minimal equipment, gets a maximum number of kids involved, and involves vigorous exercise. Kids love it. That should tell you something.

It may sound farfetched, but the discipline I learned at a young age—lifting weights under Julie's guidance—has carried through my adult life. Even the street hockey is a part of that picture. We played hard; we had rules. The karate lessons helped make me more open, more communicative, more self-confident—even though I hated going to class every week. Actually, there's a sport or exercise out there waiting for every youngster, one he or she will look forward to. You just have to find the right match. It might be something foreign to you (just look at all those soccer players), so if your boy doesn't want to be a fullback just like Dad, don't push him into it.

It is so important that we find ways of increasing the active state of mind among our young people. I regard that as the most important thing I do. In my home state of Michigan, I've been active on the Governor's Fitness Council and the Michigan Fitness Foundation. I talk to school superintendents and athletic directors. I'm working to get a coordinated fitness policy in all the schools in my home county.

We need a few hundred thousand other people pushing in the same direction.

Part Four:
Mental Discipline

22

Commitment and that Inner Fire

Knowledge alone isn't enough. If you are among the hundreds of thousands of people who have absorbed tons of good fitness information, bought gym memberships, stationary bikes and fancy shoes, and are *still* searching for a way to "stick with it," then you know—probably with painful clarity—that knowledge alone isn't enough. You are not alone. There are over-weight nutritionists and out-of-shape physiologists. There are doctors who smoke cigarettes. They all know better. What they lack is a true commitment to self, that inner fire to be the best they can be.

It all comes down to this: If you don't have that mental toughness—that inner fire—then your total fitness package will come unwrapped. Without mental discipline and a true commitment to yourself, you'll abandon your healthy new habits the second the "new" wears off, because that inner fire is what keeps it fresh and exciting. It gives you the energy to find new exercises and the discipline to push through a temporary rut.

If you read and absorb every word in this book—in a hundred books—about nutrition and exercise, all you will have gained is information. It isn't just about collecting data. For that matter, it isn't just about nutrition and exercise. It's about focusing intently on what's important and on putting one foot in front of the other in a *positive* direction—so that your steps will take you where you want to be. That applies to all three of the big ones: health and fitness, relationships, career. Most people don't focus. Their steps are aimless. And instead of living quality lives, they just exist.

I said you must train your mind in order to sustain a nutrition and exer-cise regimen. What I want to say in this section is the closest I can come to telling you how to do that. Sure, I can paint you a picture of your potential that will spark your inner fire. But I can't hand you motivational fire the way I can hand you things I know about protein and carbs and supersets. You have to reach out and develop that mental toughness yourself, because you *want* it. It's within everybody's grasp.

Most of us fight harder when we're fighting against something.

That's why what you need is within your grasp—because mistakes and adversities are the raw material to stoke your fire. If you can't find any mistakes and adversities in this world, you *really* are out of focus. Most of us find them every day. Our mistakes, other people's mistakes. Our adversities, other people's adversities. Little ones, medium-sized ones, monsters. There's enough raw material out there to turn your resolve into steel. What you need to do is take all the mistakes and adversities, grind them up and recycle them into opportunities for positive action.

Yes, we are talking about positive thinking. A constant commitment to positive thinking. I even visualize it physically in myself—I've built a transformer someplace in my gut that takes every negative ion in my body and gives it a positive charge. If you're cynical about that kind of talk, hang around a minute. Because I think the cynics are the real Pollyannas. People who have *mental toughness* have determination, that unstoppable positive attitude, the will to thrive and to confront their mistakes and adversities head-on. They don't wait for their ship to come in, *they swim out to it.*

People with a negative, "life-sucks-and-then-you-die" attitude spend their days whining and dodging the troubles they see lurking all around them. *They* are the ones who need a reality check. They may give you a hard time for not joining in on their pity party, but inside they know you are right, that you are healthier and happier for it.

Think about this: Most anyone would agree there are three big places you can have setbacks—in your health, in your personal relationships, in your finances. I had a debilitating disease that almost killed me. I had a personal relationship that left scar tissue on my heart. And then I lost nearly $200,000—virtually all my money—when my first real business deal went sour. All this by my mid-20s. But setbacks were just fuel for my fire to succeed. And now, in my early 40s, I have more energy per day than there are hours on the clock. Several businesses and several careers. A marriage with a wonderful woman who has a thousand golden attributes, and two beautiful children. Is this all an accident? No way. The gifts in my life would never have come my way if I had just given up when times got tough, instead of capitalizing on my mistakes. You could give me Yale University for Christmas and I wouldn't learn as much as I did from those three setbacks.

The mind-boggling flip side of that picture is that the world is crammed full of people who don't learn from their mistakes and adversities. Every day a few million learning opportunities get swept into the closet like dusty old textbooks. Instead of confronting them head-on with a positive-thinking mental toughness, the negative thinkers sidestep every single learning opportunity. And they land knee-deep in crud.

What do I see as an example? Here's a big one: I see a Crohn's patient a few months out of the hospital—after almost exactly the same miserable, devastating experience I went through—trying to eat pizza. Hamburgers. Hot fudge sundaes. Doritos. Beer. He comes to me for nutritional counseling, but what he really wants is a strategy for getting this stuff into his stomach. What's *wrong* with this picture? Maybe the doctors should bottle a foot or two of intestine in formaldehyde for every surgical patient and make them carry it around, just to remind them of reality.

A Crohn's patient who wants to pretend that he can knock down a beer-and-burger lunch is doing exactly what most people do with adversity in every corner of their lives, big and small. It's easier—in the short term—to shunt the problem aside, to deny it, to avoid it. And if you're a negative-thinking person, that's only logical, *because you have nothing to bring to the problem.* What's needed is to set an adversity right on the examining table, at eye level, and say: "OK, let's see what we have here and figure out what we can do with it." *That* is learning from an adversity or a mistake. *That* is the mental toughness that I wish I could bottle and give to the world. I'm not talking street-tough. I'm talking REALITY—and facing it instead of sticking your head in the sand and wishing you'd drawn a different hand.

It has to do with getting past the sorrow, the self-pity, the resentment, the temper tantrums, the "why-me" syndrome. In my case, I had to learn that a family will continue with their lives whether you are sulking in a corner or not. That your girlfriend will finally get disgusted with your negative, pessimistic personality. That the other guys on the block will get tired of hearing about your bad deck of cards and go play hockey without you. Long before Julie Levine had me looking in mirrors to check out progress on my muscles, I had to look in a mirror to check out progress on my life. Once I did that and realized that the guy staring back at me did *not* have it worse than anyone else in the universe and that he was the *only* person who could solve my problems, then I was lit. I had the spark. I was ready to try to take control of my life.

My own adversities were a blessing in disguise, because they were unavoidable monsters. The difference between having small adversities and big adversities is the difference between being in a class of 100 students and having your own personal tutor. I'll never know if I would have been smart enough to collect my advanced degree if I hadn't been told, at 15, that I might die. I'd probably be in line this afternoon at the pork shop. That's why I can say in total honesty that if I could do it all over, I wouldn't have it any other way. My life would have gone in an entirely different direction. Besides eating sausages every morning, I'd be more complacent, more naive. I'd be more cocky and self-centered. I'd have my priorities and values all screwed up. I know I wouldn't be married with a family of my own, wouldn't be thinking with as much business competency as I do.

In recent years, I've figured out that thousands of the most successful people have been blessed with serious adversity. I've met dozens of people whose health and wealth hit the top of the scale—but who also have humility, personality and a commitment to a positive lifestyle. What do they have in common? Ninety percent of them have been through some kind of trauma. They've seen both sides of the river. They learned and they remembered. They have that inner fire to make the absolute best of the life they were given.

It starts with a spark—sometimes a huge one, sometimes just a glimmer. Sparks come from a million sources. You don't have to experience trauma; you don't have to be struck by lightning. Seeing someone on the street with a smile on his face and only one leg on his body could light a spark. I know I light sparks with many low self-esteem kids when I speak at schools and explain that this muscle guy was, at their age, one very imperfect specimen. Ninety percent of the people who come to my gym for the first time are driven there by scary sparks—or by wake-up calls masquerading as sparks. A divorce, or a threat of divorce. A sudden realization of mortality. I've had first-timers come directly from the doctor's office, carrying their off-the-graph cholesterol readings.

But it takes more than a spark. It takes a strong flame, because people and events will be trying to blow out the fire every day. That is the trick to motivation, to what I am trying to pass on to you. Sparks come easy. Flames are a tougher piece of business. Most sparks are so fragile. People *want* to take control of their lives. They accumulate the knowledge and keep trying to fan the spark into a flame, but the fire never takes hold. You can't believe how many people come to me for nutrition counseling, and, after I tell them the score, say: "I *know* that." Fifty percent of their "nutrition" is coming from fat and the rest from pop and candy. I'm telling them that they're killing themselves. And they're saying: "I *know* that."

It takes much more than knowledge.

All I can conclude is that they don't really *know* anything. They've got some data stored in their head, all right, but they haven't really learned a thing. Not from their mistakes. Not from other people's mistakes. They haven't gotten a big enough wakeup call to get their attention. All this raw material going to waste. There's a level of knowledge that doesn't have anything to do with facts and numbers, and they don't have it. Live and learn? Not really. Not for most people, not most of the time.

You see, having adversity in your life isn't the secret. We all have at least some of that. Sometimes even mega-adversity or world-class mistakes aren't enough. Many people get trapped in a fail-fail-fail syndrome when the handwriting is right on the bridge of their nose. The guy with 20 straight failed relationships, for example, who says he's "still looking for the right girl." It doesn't occur to him that he should be looking in the mirror for the right *guy*—that maybe it's time for some positive change.

The secret, obviously, is the capacity to learn real-world lessons. To establish radio contact between abstract facts you "know" (excess sugar and fat are bad) and personal facts you are avoiding (you can't see your shoes). To look in a realistic mirror instead of a circus mirror that reflects only what you want to see. It's like that second lens I asked you to use when you look at the food you eat. A triple chocolate parfait sundae with whipped cream and coconut is a circus sideshow. Mega-doses of sugar, fat and cholesterol are the reality. Like the man said: "I already *know* that." But does he, really, if he's eating it? And what in the world does he see when he looks in the mirror?

We like to think that little kids live in a fantasy world and us big people are out there plowing our way through the real world. I'm not so sure. Little kids don't have to be hit by a truck to figure out that playing in the street is a bad idea. Why should you have to be diagnosed with cancer before you'll give up cigarettes? Why should you need a heart attack to truly understand what obesity and poor cardiovascular fitness can do to you? Some people need the big wakeup call. Some people have the capacity to learn.

Let me give you *my* definition of a smart person: someone who learns from *other* people's mistakes and adversities. Throw away the college entrance exams—this is a person with a mind that works in the real world. It's as simple as that. On the streets of life, he or she will play on the sidewalk instead of in the passing lane. Smart person. Am I a smart guy? I guess so, because I now learn from other people's mistakes and adversities every day. I wasn't always that smart.

Your own mistakes can be learning experiences only if they're not too big. The bigger the mistake, the more a person is likely to learn—but the more likely that it's too late.

When my Dad got sick, he talked about taking a little more time off from work, drinking less, retiring early. He decided to quit smoking, finally, and made it a point to tell me. Then he got an oxygen tank, just before the doctor called to say that Pete Nielsen had maybe a month to live. I can't tell you how hard it was to tell my Dad that his mistake was too costly. He had gotten the scare, made the commitment. But he was a day late and a dollar short. He died in *less* than a month, at 49.

Another statistic, another lesson.

If you want the whole life package, you have to start making the connections. Personally. Not in a textbook. Not in concept. *In your own life.* That's what real learning is about. We're talking permanent change. There's no quick fix. There are no substitutions on this menu. No excuses. Garbage in, garbage out. If you want to light a flame that will stay lit, then you've got to deal honestly with the only statistic you can do anything about. You. Your body, your blood pressure, your musculature, your priorities, your values. Society puts a fantasy menu in front of you every day. It's all junk food and remote controls. When you have a commitment to yourself, once you develop the discipline and mental toughness, you'll reject all of it.

"Mental toughness" sounds so macho, but it's not. Macho is fantasy— flawless and indestructible is not reality. Macho means insecurity and some kind of inferiority complex. Mental toughness means learning from mistakes, being honest with yourself. It's like tough love with yourself. You've got to sweat, but you've also got to cry. You've got to be truthful and see what's really in the mirror instead of what you'd like to see. You've got to accept that that this is the deck you've been dealt and that changes are in order. When you are mentally tough and committed to your health, you have nothing to prove. You know what you have to do. You have a game plan and you do it.

Positive thinking is the cutting edge of mental toughness. It will make you the best that you can be. And—if you are a lost, negative soul—you'll be amazed what a positive attitude can do for your relationships with other people. It only takes a minute to spread bad news. If what you project in a room—socially or at work—is pessimism, if your thinking and your conversation is dominated by what *can't* be done instead of what *can* be done, then it'll only take a minute for everybody to wish you were somewhere else.

We all like to hear good things about ourselves, and I hear two things that make me feel good. When people meet me, they say they're surprised that I'm deeper than the cosmetic look that I project (as if muscles and intelligent life couldn't co-exist). And they say that my positive outlook is *addictive* (as if anyone could get high on a negative outlook). *I'm* addicted to positive vibes in other people. Sometimes you don't even have to talk to someone to know. You can practically see the electricity. It's the opposite of the negative person. With them, you can practically hear the whine.

Do I ever get mad? Of course. Often. Do I get frustrated? Of course. Do I have negative thoughts? Thousands. I work a lot of them out in the gym.

Don't forget that one of the very biggest benefits of *physical* fitness is *mental*. You may never touch a barbell in your life, but there are other ways. All those runners you see along the road are burning more than calories. Any good exercise will do. Fitness is so good for the mind that I think I see a correlation between flabbiness and negative, angry behavior. I can't prove it, but I believe it. It *is* a package.

Positive and negative go together like love and hate. Energy is energy. You can use it positively or you can use it negatively. It's the difference between nuclear power and a hydrogen bomb. When you've got your package together, you'll always be looking to harness and channel the energy of a situation in a positive direction.

Cindy and I were at a gathering where someone dear to me collapsed with a heart attack. She turned blue. Her eyes rolled back in her head. She stopped breathing. There were 16 other guests, so there were 18 of us who were frightened and charged with energy. Sixteen people started wringing their hands and running in circles like ants on hot coals. Cindy and I helped the victim to the floor. Cindy called 911 while I started giving the victim resuscitation. Everybody had the same energy. Two of us were channeling it in a positive direction.

That's a simple, graphic example of what I mean by meeting a situation head-on, evaluating it, and deciding whether to march through it, over it, under it, or around it, choosing the most positive course. It doesn't have to be as dramatic as a heart attack. But no matter the type of obstacle—and needing to turn your physical and nutritional life around *is* an obstacle— you need to meet it head-on, one-on-one. How you respond is a *me vs. me* challenge, just like in the gym. You are the sculptor, you are in control—if you take a positive approach.

In any situation where you're scared, on the other side of scared is success. Success vs. failure is a 50/50 proposition. They're separated by such a thin line, and often that line is fear. Too many people fail even to light the flame because they're afraid they'll fall short of perfection. That's silly. It isn't about being the best in the world, or even about being the best on the block. It's about being the best you can be. No more, no less. Once the flame is lit, it's often a surprise just how good that turns out to be.

Let's say you've got the spark, and you're trying to light the flame and keep it going for the rest of your life. Let's say you've had some long conversations with yourself about making an effort to channel all your energies in a positive direction. Let's say you've done your homework, and you know a complex carbohydrate from a T-bone steak. Let's say you believe you're ready to make a commitment, but you need some training wheels. Where do you get the determination to get the thing rolling?

Focus. Focus. Focus. On what? On reality. On a specific commitment to yourself, a specific set of goals and a detailed path of how to get there. Determination comes when a person first becomes realistic and then sets realistic goals. Don't kid yourself. You've got to prioritize. If you are a couch potato, your goal isn't to win Mr. Universe next fall. Your goal might be to walk comfortably to the park and back next month.

Write down your short- and long-term goals. Make sure the time span is realistic. Don't be like the prospective clients who come to me after 30 years of abusing their bodies and expect me to make them into Venus or Adonis in 60 days. *Get real.* You've got the rest of your life to be your best. Start out by being better tomorrow than you are today—not by trying to be where you ought to be in six months or a year.

Get on a healthy diet. Get the cardiovascular system going with a modest exercise regimen like walking. Then escalate. Be better every week, every month, every year. Build your mental toughness and physical condition side by side. Accept the fact that your health is the most valuable thing you will ever have, or lose. Recognize that you are confronting the thing that people fear most: *change.* Permanent, life-altering change.

Put it all out on the table—your hopes, your fears, the reality of your fitness, where you want to be. Analyze the situation and say: "What do we have here? And what's the best way to approach it?" Don't look behind you to see who else is in the picture, because nobody can do this but you.

When you get that far, you'll start to see and hear things.

You'll get a glimpse of a determined, realistic you. That's the new you, struggling to be born.

And you'll hear a voice in your head, asking: "How *bad* do you want it?"

Get used to the voice. It'll never go away. It will be there to inspire and strengthen you at your most challenging moments. And as we walk through the final chapters, we will see how crucial it is, this new beginning that you have made. This is just the beginning of getting back on your feet. Because as you'll see next, a health and fitness lifestyle are not only rewards in themselves, helping you through each day. They are critical to helping you survive those nasty little curveballs that life will eventually throw everyone's way. Those nasty little curveballs can be major league crises—I can *personally* attest to that. By the Grace of God, a supportive family and a positive attitude, I have survived to tell the tale. Whatever your faith, don't forget the part " ... and a positive attitude." That is the key that divides the champions from the defeated.

23

The Game Plan

His words were cutting, chilling and direct: "Peter, we have problems. There is a mass the size of your fist in your abdomen, and we're not sure what it is—it could be cancer, or the Crohn's could be back. Either way, I know you are going to need surgery. We need to do some tests immediately. I need to see you first thing tomorrow morning." Those were the words of my surgeon and friend, Dr. Jason Bodzin, in February 2001.

I was in my car when I got that call. I was heading toward a relaxing evening out with my wife. Our children were home with a trusted babysitter, and I had the evening free from business commitments—businesses that revolve around fitness and health.

I was cruising down Northwestern Highway, not a care in the world. I had the sunroof open, listening to my favorite CD, enjoying an unseasonably warm and sunny February day. I was a long way from my last bout with Crohn's or any other health crisis; the days of pain, distress, and insecurity were just a faint memory. I was just enjoying life and counting my blessings.

Up until that moment, there wasn't a cloud in my sky, not a problem in my world. But as soon as I heard Dr. Bodzin's voice, I knew my world was going to change.

I turned off the music and pulled over, then Dr. Bodzin asked if I'd rather come in to his office to talk about it. "Well, now that you've got me on the edge of my seat, why don't you just lay it on me," I half-joked with him.

I guess he decided that I didn't want to waste time, because the information he gave me next had absolutely zero sugar coating.

Almost matter-of-factly he informed me that whatever the mass was, it was aggressively attacking my abdomen, and causing a life-threatening blockage of my intestine. Surgery—soon—was surely necessary to keep it from killing me. Out my car window I could see Friday afternoon traffic whiz by, as if nothing in the world had changed.

In the blink of an eye, it was like 25 years of distance from that hospital in Brooklyn had vanished. With just a few words from my doctor, I was yanked from a perfect Friday afternoon and deposited on the very familiar crossroads of life and death. Talk about a wakeup call.

When I got that call, it had been over a decade since my last bout with Crohn's disease. It had been almost 10 years since I retired from pro body-building competition after my last major world title in 1991. I had built a family and a career and a life in Michigan. They were good years—healthy, fit, busy and productive. Not without some ups and downs, but nothing nearly as painful as my first bout with Crohn's or the crash-and-burn that brought me from New York to Detroit. You could say it had been pretty smooth sailing for quite some time.

That stretch came to a screeching halt.

It was a pretty bumpy road from that February phone call to the recovery room, but each bump contained a lesson. I came out of that ordeal more mentally clear, peaceful and stronger than ever before. I was once again completely humbled by the power each of us holds in our own hands to take what looks like the worst news ever, survive it and turn it into a blessing!

How can a person be ready for a crisis? It's all about having a "game plan." No matter how healthy and fit you are, almost everyone will have to deal with a health crisis at some time in life. In this section of my story, I hope you will see yourself, and in the "game plan," a serious plan that anyone can use in order to be prepared for those inevitable health crises.

Like I have said throughout this book, a fit and healthy lifestyle can prevent a lot of health problems. But there is no *guarantee* that a health crisis won't hit you at some point in life, no matter how fit you are. In fact, my guess is that some type of health crisis, big or small, is in the cards for everyone.

So if you can't prevent health crises, why not just stick your head in the sand and hope you get lucky? Because that attitude can kill you.

We have spent a good part of this book talking about dealing with *reality*— from using that second nutritional lens to accepting where your health is right now. And we spent most of the last two parts of the book developing a "game plan" for achieving fitness. If you have put these principles into action in your life, then you are on much more solid ground regarding your health. And you are probably pulling that total package together, seeing how fitness and health require a discipline that improves your whole life.

Now we talk about another equally critical "game plan." It's the game plan for dealing with a sudden health crisis.

Health crises have had a huge impact on my life—a *positive* one, actually. As I've mentioned, my main approach to life is to take any type of adversity and turn it into opportunity—and then use it to help and teach other people. The bigger the adversity, the bigger the opportunity. Sometimes it was a physical health crisis, like the Crohn's; sometimes it was a lifestyle crisis, like business deals falling through or my "escape" from New York. Each time I took the adversity and turned it into a way to get stronger.

Along the way, I sharpened my skills at caring for my body and my mind, and focused on maintaining that "evenly yoked" lifestyle. Those roller coasters of life evened out to a huge extent. Sometimes, though, smooth sailing can make you forget that there are no guarantees. Trouble can pop up on the horizon, seemingly overnight. If some crisis comes up like that, it can yank the rug out from under your feet. *You have to know how to get back on your feet* so you can deal with the crisis.

Being prepared to deal with it is the key—and it's only possible if you have mental discipline and a seriously positive attitude.

The two weeks after that phone call were literally a battle for my life. Besides the obvious assets in that battle (such as God's help and the skill of my medical team), it came down, once again, to mental discipline—the *me vs. me* competition. I had to snap out of shock and denial and get into action, or this one was going to kill me fast. And I had to draw deep from the bank of health, fitness and mental discipline I'd built up over the years. If such a storm pops up in *your* life, how is it going to find *you?* Slumped in front of the TV or cranking it on the treadmill? Will you turn and face it or stick your head in the sand? Will you have anyone in your life to give you support? Will you *accept* it?

After the storm passed, as I looked back on those whirlwind few weeks, one thing that struck me was that it wasn't luck or chance that got me through. It was methodical, dedicated action and discipline—plus a team of people fighting with me. I looked back at all the phone calls, the doctor visits, the family meetings. The contingency planning for my businesses and personal responsibilities in my family. I could see the outline of a very methodical plan. As I recovered, comments were made about how my businesses were able to run smoothly for six weeks with minimal involvement from me—and I could see again how detailed *planning* had saved the day there as well.

Some would call me a control freak. If taking care of business so I don't die makes me a control freak, then yeah—I'm a *healthy and alive* control freak. I could also see that if I had just ignored the problem, or dissolved into a pile of self-pity, or waited for everyone else to fix it for me, there is a good chance that I wouldn't be here to tell this story.

I want to once again hold up my experiences as a mirror for you. I want you to look at my health crisis and ask yourself where you stand as far as being ready to handle something like it in your own life. I want you to see how badly it could have turned out if I hadn't had a plan for dealing with it. Why? Because I want you to learn from the experience and mistakes of others—including mine. I don't want you to learn the hard way.

Most of all, I want you to decide that part of your new health and fitness lifestyle includes a "crisis game plan"—so that *one* unavoidable crisis doesn't take away everything you've worked for.

This one unavoidable crisis had everything I'd worked for in the palm of its hand.

24

Me vs. Me

The whole thing really had begun one night earlier that month. We were having a relaxing and pleasant family evening at home. The kids were tucked into bed, my wife and I had rented a video. I was brushing my teeth and washing up before we started watching the video. Suddenly a blinding pain ripped through my abdomen, knocking me to my knees. The pain was so intense it took my breath and my vision away. Fighter instinct had me on my feet after about 30 seconds. Even though I knew inside that something was seriously wrong, the human nature in me wanted to just shake it off. The pain lasted for about 15 more seconds, and then I just finished washing up.

I leaned on the counter and looked at myself in the mirror, eye to eye. I was looking for a simple explanation for what had just happened. A hundred things went through my head: "Is this a kidney stone, maybe just gas pain? Or a pulled muscle?" Not once did I ask myself: "Is the Crohn's back?" Although that thought was knocking loud at my door.

I think in that moment, I just really didn't want to go there. Those old memories of pain and distress were just not welcome thoughts. Those days are *way* behind me ... right? Being *really* sick just isn't a part of my life anymore ... right?

On the other hand, I *know* my disease—almost as well as any doctor. I live and breathe and sleep awareness of this disease, partly because I serve as a spokesperson for the National Crohn's and Colitis Foundation of America. There is remission and there is control, but there is no cure. Yet not one time did I say to myself: "This is Crohn's. It's back."

Denial is a wonderful thing.

My wife was waiting for me downstairs, but I procrastinated in the bathroom, trying to get my head together. I finally came downstairs, and as I handed her the video, she asked me what that noise upstairs had been; she said it had sounded like a bag of bricks had hit the floor. That was me, I said. And just as I was explaining to her what had happened, it happened again, right in front of her.

The odd part is that the first thing I felt was embarrassment. I felt embarrassed in front of my wife, to whom I'd been married 11 years, who has been through many ups and downs with me and stood by me through it all. But I am supposed to be the strong one, the provider for the family. To my wife and children, I'm Superman, their rock. And I didn't want to let my wife see her rock crumbling! Pride can stay intact through a lot of pain.

Cindy wasn't worried about my pride—and logically she wanted to call 911. We know that the No. 1 rule when someone goes down is: "Call 911 and ask questions later." But my pride jumped in and said: "No way! We are *not* calling 911!" So she immediately called our family doctor and friend, Dr. Marshall Sack.

I knew that the responsible thing to do was run this episode by the doctor, even though at some level I just wanted to forget that it had happened. But years of mental training to deal with things head-on wouldn't let me stick my head in the sand like that. Key point—you *have* to deal with it—even if you don't feel like it. So I talked to Dr. Sack.

He asked me lots of "doctor" questions about the pain—where it was located, how long it had lasted, that kind of thing. After a detailed conversation, he told me that it was probably just a pulled muscle, but that I would need to get in to his office if it continued. I knew deep down that it was organ pain, not muscle pain, but I was too tired to argue. Besides, I *wanted* him to be right; wouldn't it be nice if it were just a pulled muscle? Those old dusty memories of the Crohn's were starting to get clearer, and I didn't like it.

He told me to get in for an exam with a specialist the next day. I was exhausted by that time, so I hung up the phone and Cindy and I went to bed.

The next morning I phoned my close friend and surgeon, Dr. Bodzin, a specialist of the intestinal tract, stomach and esophagus. He's also a specialist in Crohn's disease. Looking at my chart, he spoke to me over the phone and said: "I don't like the way this sounds, Peter. You haven't been in for an exam in four years. It's time to do another checkup. Come in this morning."

That got my attention.

He did a sigmoidoscopy, a check of the lining of the last three feet of the large intestine. I'd been having this checkup as a standard Crohn's patient procedure every few years, with perfect results. That day the results looked good again, but Dr. Bodzin's sharp eye and instincts caught a little redness, so he ordered biopsies. He also ordered a colonoscopy, a blood test and a lower and upper GI. For those of you not familiar with the procedure, it's pretty much the most invasive stem-to-stern checkup you can possibly have, and I personally would prefer a two-hour beating. But I wanted to stay alive more than I wanted to cater to my pride, so I agreed. Again, you *have* to deal with it, whether you feel like it or not.

Men, are you listening? We are the kings of avoiding health exams, especially the invasive ones. Are you willing to die for your pride?

So off I went to that humbling medical experience.

I was feeling fine after that day—no more pain. I followed through with the exams and pretty much forgot about the whole thing after a day or two. It sort of "went away" in my mind. I got absorbed in the energy, challenge and joy that is my everyday life. No more pain, no more problem. The rest of the week went by and I cruised into that pleasant Friday afternoon on my way to that date with my wife. All was well. And then I got my wakeup call.

I would love to tell you that I had a perfect reaction, that I just hung up the phone and clicked right in to "deal with it" gear, ignoring the devastation I felt inside. But what I had instead was a *perfectly normal* reaction—fear, denial, anger and, yes, a bit of self-pity for Mr. Health and Positive Thinking.

I hung up the phone, and clicked down a pretty normal reaction list:

• **Fear and Denial.** "Oh God, not again. This isn't happening. Maybe Dr. Bodzin is wrong. I need a second opinion."

• **Anger and Self-pity.** "This is going to get in the way of my life, damn it! I don't have time for this! This is not what I had planned! Ten years in complete remission, regular checkups, a meticulously healthy diet and a world-class fitness regimen. I did *everything right!* How can this be happening?"

• **Bargaining.** "OK. Suppose it's true. I can put off surgery for two months, finish my appearance tour, record my television and radio shows in advance, and finalize the deal on my new club. Then I'll deal with it."

I drove down that highway in my own personal hell for about 10 minutes. I call it my personal hell, because my head was filled with anger, self-pity and denial, and to me, nothing is more painful (or dangerous) than that state of mind. Those feelings are a normal part of dealing with really bad news, but left unchecked, they rob you of precious moments of life. They can distract or even prevent you from taking action to help yourself. They are like thieves, stealing whatever chance you have to turn bad news around. You have to be ready to recognize it when you get in this space— no one can do it for you, and you sure aren't going to listen to anyone else tell you about it. Mental discipline and self-honesty is the only way—you have to get in your own face and get real with yourself.

My hands were almost numb on the steering wheel. I felt myself starting to spiral down. Then I remembered two things: my mental discipline and my faith.

First, my mental discipline and attitude kicked in: "Whoa. Stop this line of thinking right here. This is NOT how winners think. If this is a catastrophe, then it has a twin: opportunity. No way am I going to just lay down and die."

Second, my faith kicked in: "You don't have to handle this all by yourself. In fact, you can't. So hand it over to Someone who can." And I did. It was just that simple for me, after years of practice at "handing it over."

It's like I could instantly feel my hands on the steering wheel again. I was flooded with an incredible sense of relief and peace, because I knew two things if I knew nothing else: First, I am going to do everything in my power to face this thing and pull out all the stops to win. Second, God is on my side. Together, we are going to tackle this and win. I gripped the steering wheel of my car—and of my life. That familiar inner fire was lit— not just a spark—a strong flame, all the way through my soul.

It's not like I got happy about it; I was not *ready* to hear the news. But I was *willing* and *prepared* to deal with it, and that is why I am here today to tell you about it. I could have stuck my head in the sand and temporarily avoided the pain I felt. Of course, in my case, I could have been dead within two weeks. I could have wasted more precious time being angry and refusing to deal with it, with the same results. Thanks to God and mental training, I didn't do either. By now you know I love a good challenge, and the battle was on.

25

You Gotta Have a Plan

I am convinced that the most dangerous time in handling a crisis is when a person is still in shock from bad news. Will they just get stuck in shock and stay paralyzed, or will they launch into action to help themselves? How will *you* react at the moment of truth? How will *you* deal with the personal crisis that will inevitably come your way? Knowing that about yourself is critical to having a "game plan" for dealing with health crises.

I'm not just talking about the crisis of Crohn's disease, or cancer, or diabetes or other dread diseases. A health crisis can take the form of poor results from your annual physical. Or realizing that you are overweight and severely out of shape. It can be a substance abuse problem like smoking or drinking, a serious injury, or the loss of a loved one through death or divorce. The point is, a health crisis can be mental, physical or emotional. It is a moment when it seems that someone pulled the rug out from under your life. Even if the nature of your crisis is different from mine, we human beings have a lot in common in the way we feel and react to loss. Therefore, we can help each other, which I feel is my true purpose in life.

Your life might be the perfect picture of smooth sailing right now ... I am talking to *you!* Don't get caught so off guard by a future crisis that you pay the ultimate price! Even if you have no crises in your life right now, know that as a human being there will inevitably be one on the horizon for you or someone you love. And if you are currently dealing with a health crisis, or recently did but are struggling with the results, a lot of this is going to sound very familiar to you. You *must* have a game plan to deal with a crisis, or *it* will deal with *you.*

Finding out that I had some unknown monster wreaking havoc in my gut felt like someone had pulled the rug out from under me—but I knew I had to make a plan and get with the program, or this monster was going to call all the shots.

My game plan saved my life.

Like most people, I get the best results by working on things a piece at a time, so my game plan is split into seven simple steps. My hope is that you will see yourself in how I reacted to my situation and will be able to benefit from my experience. It is my goal that everyone sees that they have the power to manage a crisis instead of being managed by it and to turn a health catastrophe into an opportunity.

Here is the basic outline of my "Game Plan."

1. Prepare Yourself Now.
2. Don't Run. Get the Facts.
3. Stay Calm. Take Care of the Basics.
4. Assemble Your Team.
5. Chart Your Course.
6. See It Through.
7. Seize the Miracle.

So far, this book has been all about step one—Prepare Yourself Now. I have to talk about that step first thing, because it is so wrapped up in the decision to go on with the rest of the steps. We'll go into the nuts and bolts of steps two through seven in the next couple of chapters.

If you are *still* asking yourself why you should be concerned with any of this, if you think you'd rather just go on in blissful ignorance of what the future holds, it's basically like refusing to save for retirement because you're not sure how much you'll need—or if you'll make it that long. Let me give you some more motivation.

As I've said, there was a lot of living between my early years in the Motor City and the day I found out I was sick again. I had married, launched a successful business and started a family. My family is the absolute center of my life. I walked what I talked in the pages of this book, seeking the most I could get from my health, my life and myself, and making it useful to my family and to others.

I experienced continued success with my personal training club, as well as my nationally syndicated television and radio shows, several exercise videos, an active Web site (www.peternielsen.com), and tons of appearances. I have such deep gratitude for the life I have had the privilege to build—especially considering my humble and frail beginnings.

I also continued to be active in volunteer work for the Crohn's and Colitis Foundation of America (www.ccfa.org) as one of their national spokespersons. As much as I try to give in that role, it always seems like helping others with Crohn's helps me as much as it helps them. Anytime I give of myself, it has a healing effect on my whole soul.

During that decade, I expanded my spiritual life, too. I developed close friendships within my church, gaining a great friend, Darryl Wood, who also has become my spiritual guide. My friendships and family are what keep my feet on the ground. When I have to sort out something really big, I look for spiritual guidance from Darryl, and in prayer with God. I also turn to my family and friends—my wife Cindy, and my best friend Tom Celani, who is like a brother to me.

And, of course, I continued to maintain peak physical training and nutrition. It's just how I believe in caring for the one and only fragile frame that God gave me. Plus, I pretty much make my living by being a walking example of the fitness lifestyle. My life has continued to revolve around all of the things we talked about: exercise, nutrition, discipline and quality living.

All of this adds up to a pretty healthy guy—physically, mentally, spiritually, emotionally and financially. And I *still* got hit with a crisis! I thought that living healthy and right meant no more crises!

I was wrong.

The week before my Crohn's relapse, I had just crated and shipped my Harley to Florida. I was planning to meet it and my best friend, Tom, for a series of Florida appearances, adding in some bike cruising and fishing in the Keys. On top of that, the ink was barely dry on contracts to expand my fitness clubs. As I said before, there was not a cloud in my sky!

What will *you* do if you have worked all your life, now you're the CEO, you have the big house, the sports cars, the expensive suits, or maybe you're just happy with your latest promotion, the nice 401(k) nest egg, the two cars and the nice vacations—then ... wham! There is no amount of power or success that will insulate you from an unexpected crisis! And I *personally* can vouch for that!

What I was doing didn't *prevent* my crisis, but no doubt the cards were stacked in my favor due to my lifestyle. I was getting regular checkups for the Crohn's—which meant every couple of years, for my length of remission. My training and nutrition lifestyle meant that my body was in the best possible condition to handle any curveballs that life decided to throw. My friendships and faith ensured that I kept the right mental attitude and kept my ego in check, which promotes level-headed and healthy thinking—another insurance policy for handling those curveballs. I was taking care of business with my whole self. Everything we've talked about in this book.

And that *foundation* was key in my survival. This is the point when I ask you, are you taking care of business with *your* whole person? Where are your friendships? Do you have a solid emotional support team for good times and bad? Are you taking care of yourself—with good nutrition, exercise and regular checkups? Or are you gulping down fast food four or five times a week and watching 15-plus hours of TV a week?

I'm ringing the warning bell for *you*, because when the crisis comes knocking at your door, I hope it finds you in peak condition with a life full of healthy, positive people. I pray that it doesn't find you zoned out in front of the TV with a cheeseburger in one hand and a cigarette in the other. If you are making a great living and are on top of the world, know that you are not prepared if you are guzzling booze in your first class airline seat and the farthest you ever walk is out to your luxury car. The wallet is only a thin shield.

I am alive today because when the knock came on my door, I was standing on a firm foundation in a house of bricks. And it was *still* tough for me! Don't be standing on sand in a house of sticks when the hurricane comes.

26

Getting Ready for Battle

So you've decided that you want to hold on to what you're working so hard for, even if some crisis deposits itself in your lap tomorrow—or next month, next year, or in 10 years. Let's dive right in to the game plan. For those of you who are chapter-surfers, we'll start with a recap of the first step of the plan:

STEP ONE—PREPARE YOURSELF NOW

Basic (but serious) self-maintenance is the first key. It is the same healthy lifestyle we have spent most of this book discussing. As you know by now, preparation does not mean you have to run a marathon or win a fitness contest or eat only seeds and nuts and raw vegetables. It means you know where your health stands today and you are actively involved in pursuing reasonable, healthy goals to improve or maintain it. You use that second nutritional lens for food and you get regular exercise. Mental discipline at the breakfast, lunch and dinner table, and on the way to your workout, is part of *who you are* now.

This step isn't something you'll really "finish," it's something you will do every day as part of a healthy lifestyle. You'll get better and better at it every month and every year. It's the bank you'll build up over time, and when a crisis hits you, you'll withdraw as much as you need from that fitness account. Fit people recover better—from surgeries, disease, accidents and most types of trauma. *Markedly* faster and better than people who smoke, have lousy diets, or are just plain couch potatoes.

So the key here is keep up with everything you've learned so far in this book. Eat right and stay active.

Preparation does not mean that you get to completely avoid hard times, but you will cut out the preventable ones and will be in peak shape to respond to the ones you can't avoid. I had quite the curveball thrown at me, and I had to call in every single healthy trump card that my disciplined lifestyle had bought me.

STEP TWO—DON'T RUN. GET THE FACTS.

This step is basically about acting better than you feel. Mental discipline. Your thoughts are your own and can't directly hurt you. But thoughts lead to feelings, which lead to action (or inaction). I'm not talking about all the random thoughts that constantly stream through your head on any given day. I'm talking about the conversations you have with yourself—in your head—about things that count. I give myself a break for the first couple answers I come up with when I'm faced with serious problems. Sometimes you have to wait to act until level-headed thinking kicks in.

For example, when I hung up the phone in my car, my surgeon had just told me that he had discovered a life-threatening condition and he was prepared to act on it immediately to save my life. What *I* heard was: "Peter, I have found something in your abdomen that means you have to put your entire life on hold; forget all the important things you want to do right now, forget all your plans. *You have no choice.*"

All I could think about was the things I was going to have to give up if I listened to this guy—you know, the board-certified surgeon at a nationally ranked hospital, but what does he know? I broke into a dead run, mentally. You are probably thinking: "But if you don't take care of the issue, don't you stand to lose much more, like your life?" Exactly. If you don't take care of business, you stand to lose your life. It's as simple as that.

But the mind is a wonderful thing. It tries to protect us from trauma with all kinds of clever devices, one of which is the big D: denial. You can't prevent an initial reaction of denial, but you must own it and manage it before it starts managing you.

Denial will tell you to think only about the replaceable things you might lose, such as money, career opportunities or prestige. It lets you hide from what you might really lose—like your life and time with your family. Or it will tell you to forget about it, that just thinking about it is going to be too painful to handle. So you just shut down.

My only response to Dr. Bodzin on that phone call was: "Are you sure?" Lucky for me, he is far too experienced of a professional to be insulted when I question him like that. He recognizes shock when he sees it.

The dubious "plus" side of denial is that you can pretend that you can make a problem go away by refusing to deal with it—and actually talk yourself into believing it! The minus side of that coin is that untended problems *always* get worse. It's like when you get bills in the mail that you are afraid you can't pay, so you leave them unopened on the counter—or quit going to the mailbox altogether. In my experience, no one ever forgot my debts. And my debts never miraculously reversed themselves. Unpaid debts are always in the back of your mind. The escape of denial is a *total* illusion.

I have no other way to say it: You just have to face the monster, whatever it is. Grab it with both hands, look it in the face and lean into it. That is mental toughness, and you have to build it like a muscle over time. (None of us ever has to do that alone, so keep reading!)

Now for me, facing the beast was a piecemeal job, done over a couple of days. Once you grab that beast to face it, remember that you don't have to take it down all in one fell swoop. That will just overwhelm you. Take it piece by piece. Start by *making the decision* that you are going to face it. It may sound basic, but so many people never even get that far. You have accomplished a lot when you have made the decision: "I am going to *deal* with this—I'm not sure *how*, but I *am* going to deal with it."

I made the decision in my car to face it, and I turned to my faith and my mental discipline to strengthen me for the fight. Despite the human urge to just run, I decided to see the doctor, look at the test results and listen to what he had to say. That's all. It doesn't even mean that I had to believe him yet! A piece at a time, remember?

You can do the same thing, too. Write it down if you have to. Even if you have to tell yourself that this is all you're going to do, at least get the facts.

I didn't tell Cindy about the situation that night during our dinner date, or even the next morning before I went to the doctor. I know, I know ... how could I not tell my life's partner? Because taking this to my wife would make it real for both of us. Saying out loud to her: "The Crohn's is back, and I need surgery to stay alive," would mean, first, that I turn her world upside down, too, and second, that there would be no turning back from dealing with it. It's a personal decision, but you can't keep your family in the dark for long—it's not fair to them or you.

The second big piece of facing it was when I showed up at the doctor's office the next morning. You make a great step in *deciding* to get the facts. Now you have to take that next step, and actually show up and get them!

I listened and watched as Dr. Bodzin showed me the insides of my gut on an MRI. There was an undeniable mass. Worse, my ileum (the lower small intestine, where much absorption of certain vitamins and nutrients occurs) was reduced to the diameter of a shoestring, along a length of about 12 inches. The *normal* inner diameter would be about that of a small garden hose. This is classic Crohn's symptomology, where ulcerations caused by the disease appear in the intestinal wall, then leave scar tissue behind. The scar tissue narrows the intestinal pathway, causing partial or complete obstruction of intestinal flow, which creates a growing bulge of backed-up digestive material. Nice, huh? I basically had a volcano of toxic material in a fragile sac in my abdomen, and when it blew, I could be dead of toxic shock within 20 minutes.

I left Dr. Bodzin's office appearing ice-cool and calm. No one passing me in the parking lot would have known the weight on my mind. We all feel that we have to stay strong and keep it all together, don't we? But by the time I got to my car, it was all I could do to get inside and close the door before I leaned my head and arms on the steering wheel and just let myself "break down" for a while.

Let me say a little something about a healthy "breaking down" session. I have some world bodybuilding titles and I can bench press, curl and lift a lot of poundage. But to build all those muscles, I first have to break them all down with resistance training and then build them back up with nutrition and rest. Without that constant cycle of breaking down and building up, your muscles will just atrophy as time goes on, leaving you weaker with each passing year. Same goes for your "heart" muscle—I mean the figurative one, not the actual one that pumps blood through your body. Letting yourself break down and *feel* is definitely part of the total package of a healthy lifestyle. For your "emotional heart" to be strong, you have to let those hard times come and weigh on it, and you have to let it break down a little before you can rebuild it. When you do, it will be stronger and more whole than before. The fact that I can break down and cry, that I can allow myself to feel sad or even afraid, I now see as one of my most *important* strengths. Some of that I get by nature—I have always been a passionate person. Some of it I get by having a wife and children—if you can't feel, you can't really share their life. You might dam up your feelings at the beginning of a crisis, but eventually you have to let them flow through you like a river and clean you out. Hold them in too long and the dam will break—usually creating a lot of carnage through anger, directed at all the wrong people.

That was the third piece—don't run *emotionally*, either.

Not running away does not equal inaction. While you are doing such a great job of not running, stay in motion to gather all the facts. Make sure you fully understand and believe your situation. With stakes that high (your health, your life), you need to get *all* of the facts.

In my case, I wanted a second opinion.

I got back on the phone, and arranged for a second opinion. (Like I said, I may need to question, but I don't waste time.) I have never believed in anyone or anything that I couldn't question. I questioned my diagnosis, the facts, even my doctor and friend, Jason Bodzin. I got an independent reality check from another fine doctor and basically confirmed what I knew in my heart. Surgery was necessary. It is absolutely critical you believe that your situation is real. It will let you move forward without doubts so you can participate without hesitation in your own recovery.

You will still find opportunities to fall into denial at every step. I had one doctor telling me that, yes, I definitely needed surgery, that my first diagnosis was correct, but that he could try to manage my condition for eight weeks, so that I could go to Florida, make my appearances, launch my new venture ... I had to laugh when I heard that, because a top-notch, well-intentioned doctor was telling me exactly what that sneaky little Denial troll inside me was hoping to hear. And out loud, it sounded ridiculous. Sometimes it just takes hearing someone else feeding a ridiculous plan back to you to really see just how ridiculous it is. People will try to give you what you push for. You can absolutely risk your life so that you won't have to miss part of the parade—and no one will stop you! I thanked the doctor genuinely and went back to contact my primary doctors.

At that point, I felt a ton of bricks fall off my shoulders, because I had stopped fighting against it, stopped trying to deny it, and stopped trying basically to strike a bargain with God. You can fight your situation, but not forever. You can deny reality, but it will eventually catch you. You can put off dealing with it, but when your time is up, *it* will deal with *you* instead.

Fighting and running will just pile so much extra weight onto your shoulders. Please don't hold on to it for too long. Besides missing the peace that comes from letting go, you may pay the ultimate price of your life. I just had to let it go.

When I did, I dialed Dr. Bodzin and scheduled the surgery. And would you believe it? He had already scheduled three surgery dates for me, postponing his vacation, hoping I would come to my senses in time for the first date and in time to save my life. I thank God for him, and will never forget how he stood and waited, patient and unshakable. Like a father.

How tragic it would have been, had I been on the road or on a plane when this thing inside me blew up. If I had just so *happened* to be near an emergency room when it exploded, I *may* have survived—but I would not have had my choice of surgeons, much less someone familiar with my case. If I had survived, which is unlikely, I would have risked massive and unnecessary muscle damage from the knife, blood transfusions, as well as a hurried epidural, which can leave lasting back pain. My muscles and my back are a big part of my living! What are *you* willing to risk just so that you won't have to change your plans? Some scars? The ability to walk? Your life?

So for me, "Don't Run" means that I turn and face the truth head-on, even if I have to break it into pieces and chew them one at a time. Remember, you are allowed to break it down so that you can drink the truth from a glass instead of from a fire hose.

STEP THREE—STAY CALM. TAKE CARE OF THE BASICS.

Are you old enough to remember watching Godzilla movies? The creators were smart—they knew how to invoke our deepest fears. Here was this huge, horrible monster, bigger than anything we had ever seen, and way stronger than any weapon we had. It was angry, hungry and had no mercy. Not even the police or army could do anything. Even if you ran, you never knew when he was going to peel back the roof of your house and eat you like a banana.

It sounds like the way many people initially picture a crisis.

If you remember those movies, you know how the people reacted: Most of them ran screaming through the streets like a bull run gone bad—trampling one another, out of their minds with fear. A cop takes a shot at the beast, which was as effective as throwing a BB at a semi truck to slow it down. Then he got snatched up and swallowed as a reward for his efforts. Not a hopeful picture. And did some superhero come along and save us? Did Godzilla ever decide he was done with us and lumber off to the sea and just disappear? Nope.

The solution was always to calmly face the beast with a well-thought-out plan of attack based on logic, science and teamwork. Lots of mental discipline and well-planned action.

You have to *plan* the same way—with logic, facts and teamwork—when confronting a crisis.

When I fully understood, believed and accepted that my Crohn's was back, I calmly took care of the basics of my life. Here is what they may look like for you:

- Tell your spouse or life's partner. (At this point, I told Cindy.)

- Tell your best friend. (For me, this was Tom.)

- Talk with your spiritual guide, pastor or "life" mentor. (I talked with my pastor and with Darryl, who helped me accept that this was part of a plan that I did not yet understand—*stay focused.*)

- Talk to God, or whatever Higher Power that makes sense and brings you comfort and direction, or at least to your best mentor. (I told God that I had some fear, but was ready for whatever He had planned.)

- Continue to get adequate sleep and exercise and tighten your nutrition. You are preparing for battle, and your body must be ready. (I also increased my water intake to help my body eliminate toxins. A crisis is not an excuse to binge-eat or drink; in fact, those things would have been the ultimate mistake for me!)

- Don't let any of the other basics go downhill. You still have to get up, shower and eat right. If OK'd by your doctor, exercise too. It's called "suiting up and showing up." (I still made my bed, obeyed the speed limit, went to work and said my prayers. Crisis is no excuse to develop bad habits or let go of good ones.)

And because this was a serious situation and I am responsible for my family, I put my affairs in order to ensure that a life without me would be financially comfortable for my wife and children. You may not want to think about it, but picture a family that is not only grieving, but also broke. Get that kind of worrying off your plate or it will put a dent in your focus.

With your ship in shape, you are on top of step three. Now you need a crew to help you man the battleship.

STEP FOUR—ASSEMBLE YOUR TEAM

No world champion ever gets to the top alone, myself included. Earlier I told you about my first core fitness team: Julie Levine, my Dad, My Mom and Yvonne. Even though the team members have changed over the years, I have always had a support team and been a member of others' support teams. My permanent support team includes my wife, my friends Tom and Darryl, my mother, my pastor, and, of course, God as head coach. Plus a couple of business mentors. Who is *your* core support team? Could you call them all in right now, today, to help you through a crisis? Are their phone numbers written down? Are you current with them? Would *you* support *them?*

As captain of your support team, it is *your* responsibility to make sure that the people you bring into your life are a positive influence, to whom your well-being is important. That is getting into the "total package" of a healthy lifestyle. If you pick the right people, they will go to the wall for you. I am the orchestrator of my response team, so I *know* I can count on my people.

Look at it this way. You may let a stranger cut your lawn, but you sure won't let a stranger watch your children.

When my crisis came up, I called in all my team members and we went into a huddle (actually, a series of conference calls). My support team is a mixture of people who are my friends, mentors and collaborators, each with their own area of expertise:

- The physical, medical and surgical team players. Dr. Jason Bodzin, Dr. Marshall Sack, and Dr. Michael Duffy. They assembled their own world-class surgical team and took responsibility to repair the damage and do no harm. When you are dealing with a crisis, your health is your own responsibility, so pick these people well.

- The logistical team players. My wife, Cindy, and my club managers, John Bonner and Anita Gandol. Together, they basically keep my training club world running. Your spouse may have to temporarily take over the house and help you organize a lot of what is going to happen. Who are your colleagues or co-workers? You must find at least one trusted person at your work who is willing to watch over some of your details, so that you don't come back to a train wreck.

- The emotional support team players. Cindy, Tom and Darryl. These are the people who love me inside and out and have stood beside me through the best and worst of times. They are the people in front of whom I can truly be me, the people I lean on the heaviest. These people are going to be closest to you during your toughest moments. You *must* let yourself lean on them—the fear at some moments may be so great that you channel it into anger and direct it at your inner circle. Don't make that mistake! Just do your best to vent your fears with your inner circle and let them in—so you don't lash out and lose them. My team may not be perfect at all times, but they are perfectly loyal to me, and that is a gift beyond price.

- The spiritual team. My wife, Darryl, my church pastor, Calvin Ratz, and God. With this team, I shore up my faith. Whether you are religious, or have fallen away from a faith that works for you, or are agnostic or an atheist—it never hurts to have as many people rooting for you as possible. Whether they are praying for you, thinking of you, or just talking to each other about wishing you well, it is my firm belief that this collective goodwill helps. Religious or not, positive energy and goodwill have an amazing amount of power to heal.

- Business/financial team. Accountant, lawyer and managers. Allies like Rick Agree have always kept my creative ideas firmly rooted in fiscal reality. Turn to this group of people to safeguard your financial goals and fiscal responsibilities to family, employees and the government in your absence. Deals will get made and people must get paid, even if you're on your back in the hospital.

The point is you don't ever have to go through a crisis alone—in fact, you shouldn't! I could have chosen to revert to my old "lone wolf" self—but it would have been the worst possible timing. Some of us have a first instinct to fold it all in and go it alone. If you get to your crisis point and find you have no such team, then get busy. In the middle of a crisis is not the best time to have to find your allies—but it can definitely be done, and it beats going it alone. I knew without a doubt that I needed as much help as I could get. Hope and optimism alone were not going to fix the complicated mess in my abdomen.

Notice that I did not have some random set of support people that I pulled out of the phone book. I had been working with my people for years, and they all have repeatedly stood the test of time—and my questioning. When it comes to your family and your life, don't do anybody any favors at your expense. You only want people by your side who are committed, talented, skilled and prepared. That may sound cold, but it's survival. And it's your responsibility. Save the risk-taking for lower stakes.

There was one last, unplanned piece left for assembling my team. So far, I had kept the news of my crisis confined within my inner circle of support and family. I had sort of forgotten that I am nationally and locally recognized; my frequent public appearances and radio and television shows mean that I am often recognized and approached in public, which is always a pleasure. People want to talk fitness and motivation, my favorite subjects, and there is always that curiosity people have about what a television personality is really like in person. I figured that people were more interested in my strengths and successes—in what I can share about fitness and health. Why would people be interested in my struggles or my shortcomings? People would just be disappointed if they had to see me in anything but top form, right?

Wrong!

I would later be amazed, post-recovery, at the number of people who came up to me in public to ask how I felt. Not to ask me about a lifting technique or for a training or nutrition tip. They wanted to know how *I* was.

So I had a decision in front of me about just how private I wanted to keep my crisis. You may not want people to know you are struggling. You may not want them to see that you are in crisis and that you need help. Many of us have this "Superman" thing going on, and we don't want the world to see our kryptonite. Sometimes the best thing that can happen to take that weight off your shoulders is to have someone else "blow it" for you! God made the decision for me. In my case, losing my "privacy" turned out to be a huge therapeutic experience.

See, I was pretty committed to the idea of keeping my crisis totally private. I had decided that my health and fitness level are a big part of my living, and that going public could mean I'd lose it all. (A little tunnel vision there.) Yet I could see and feel the tremendous burden this "secret" placed on my shoulders. So when, without my knowledge, the news of my condition went public, it turned out to be another blessing.

I had my privacy under wraps until someone "blew it"—to the press. Luckily I got a warning shot that this was going down. Not only was it a personal matter, it was a business matter for me—I have contractual obligations with my television and radio producers regarding news stories about my life.

God's plans were different from mine, and as always, His turned out better. I got the message: "Let it all go, Peter. I own your muscles, your health and your success. I didn't bring you this far to drop you on your head now. Get out of the way so I can bring better things to you, and better things to others, through you." The privacy was over.

If you pay attention, these "surprises" are really God acting through others. Are you willing to let the world see your struggle in the event that it may help other people?

I immediately called Deborah Collura, the news director at WDIV-TV (NBC in Detroit). I explained the situation to her and set up a meeting with herself and Bob Ellis, who at that time was the special projects manager (he later became the assistant news director). Bob had already become a great friend and amazing collaborator for my TV shows. We brought in John Pompeo, the best cameraman I personally know. I opened my heart and my story to this phenomenal team, and they became great collaborators and friends to me. Later I will share more about the incredible time we shared putting together the prime time television special that chronicled my health crisis and recovery. (That television special went on to win an Emmy!)

You may not be worried about reporters exposing every detail of your crisis to the world. But if it makes you feel completely naked and exposed to know that other people know what is going on with you during a crisis, you know the feeling I had. It is just one more chunk of letting go during a huge crisis. It doesn't matter if it is the syndicated press or the family grapevine that blows your cover. It is all about *your* acceptance in the end.

This is where you will get a peek at the one of the deepest lessons a crisis has to offer. We talked about being prepared, getting support, assembling your team. All of those things got you closer to understanding the bigger picture. The bigger picture is all about surrender.

When I was wrapping my mind around this whole situation, at each step I learned more about what I could and couldn't do. Letting everyone know about the crisis I faced was my last surrender, because I thought for sure it meant the end of my career. What is the last thing you will surrender?

Think of the things you hold most dear, after your family: career, physical ability, looks, money. Now picture letting them go to save your life and your family. I had to be willing to put it all in God's hands, to accept that if He wanted to take my career, my muscles, and my strength, and break me all the way down to putty, then they were His to take, and I had to trust in Him for the outcome. Either I was going to trust Him, or I wasn't. You don't have to be religious or wrap your surrender around God to get this point. It is all about taking control of the right things and letting the rest go. Listen for that quiet voice inside telling you to let go, whether you call it God, or good conscience, or whatever. The reward of paying attention to it is an incredible sense of peace. I listened, and when I was obedient the rush of relief came.

I had never had so much to lose, and when I finally surrendered it was the most liberating act of my life.

Once you have assembled your team, you are ready to make your detailed survival plan.

27

Charting Your Course

By now you have accepted whatever crisis has been dumped in your lap. You have the facts, you understand them, and you're willing to deal with it. You've gotten your inner circle of support together. You have decided that one way or another, you are going to come out on top of this situation. It's "when" you get through it, not "if." Getting through it is officially a project.

This is where pure methodical planning is your best friend.

STEP FIVE—CHART YOUR COURSE

Your crisis management team is in place and you have a clear knowledge of where you stand right now; it's time to set *specific* goals and chart *exactly* how you are going to get from point A to point B, a full recovery. Without proper planning, the most talented team in the world will falter.

Dr. Bodzin put together his own A-list surgical team. He tapped a world-class anesthesiology and nursing team. They charted out every turn of a very technical procedure and rehearsed the surgery like a scrimmage before the big game. How do I know that? I checked! That's right—I checked what my team was doing, and you should, too. The project they are working on is your life, so you have the ultimate right to "butt in"!

Your team will take its cue for how hard to work for you from how hard you work for yourself. I participated as a key team member by keeping my body well and being up on all the facts of my case. At the very least, you should deliver to your team a body that is in the best possible physical and nutritional condition, well-rested and well-hydrated.

You will need a blueprint for how you are going to carry out the details of daily life, if you will not be fully in the picture for a short (or long) while.

In my case, I was going to be in the hospital for a few days and then at home for six weeks. At the helm of logistics and emotional support is my wife, Cindy. Remember me telling you that I am the rock of my family? Well, it turns out that Cindy is my rock, too. She very efficiently kept our home and private affairs running, and got the house ready for my six-week hiatus.

Who is *your* rock? You must talk to that person ahead of time and make a plan for all the things that he or she will have to take over for you. My personal commitments and my business run like precision machines, thanks in large part to Cindy. Together with my club managers, we captured all the details of how they would handle my daily personal duties at home and the office while I was recovering. You will need to sit down with pencil and paper with these folks and plan, plan, plan. Plan everything from who will return your voice mail and email to who will take out the trash. Details, details, details. They are *key* to a smooth recovery.

I also made a plan to continue my spiritual practices before, during and after surgery. I met with Darryl and Pastor Ratz to sharpen my focus and my faith in God. We made a plan to meet during my home recovery phase. This planning will help your spirit stay strong while you recover. Again, it doesn't *have* to be a church thing to be effective. It can be your family or even your Harley buddies. Think of it as your booster team.

The last area where you need to make plans is in your business affairs. I cannot emphasize enough the importance of making these plans, because if you don't manage it up front, it will dog you when you most need your energy focused on the crisis itself. Bills have to be paid, right? You're going to get through this, right? Therefore, you want the least possible hassle from business affairs during your recovery.

This planning starts now, when you are not in a crisis. If you run a sloppy business, it's tough enough to keep up during normal circumstances. If you leave it sloppy, or worse yet, don't make plans to manage an absence during a crisis, you may live to regret it. What if paychecks don't go out and bills go unpaid? No, it's not the end of the world. But I refuse to let a crisis come through my life like a tornado. I have some control there.

If you work for a big company, you may think you don't care, but the effects always show up. The first thing that will happen is that there will be a huge backlog stressing you out when you are trying to focus on recovery. You have to plan so that you can allow yourself to be out of control of the details for a while and let people you trust be in control, using a plan you made together. It's called sharing the load. It may be the first time you are forced to do it—who knows, maybe that's the whole purpose of what the crisis will teach you.

I put in many extra hours before my surgery to pre-record my television and radio shows and get payroll out in advance. I had picked the early surgery date so I could get released from the hospital before the next pay period and do the next payroll from home. It may sound extreme, but it is all part of following a game plan and not letting your entire life unravel because of a temporary crisis.

If you plan like a fiend the way I did, you may be amazed at how well your life runs without you! I learned growing up that I had to take care of business because no one could take care of it for me. Unfortunately, many of us also learned some not-so-good things that make it hard to trust people with our affairs. I had never spent more than two days away from my business, because I am so focused and, well, controlling. I'm sure my staff would agree. I am very driven and detailed, and my businesses run like a well-oiled machine. What I realized during my hiatus was that my team could run it with their eyes closed. The payoff was that I was out for six weeks, and my business continued to thrive in my absence. In fact, my people were free to try out some ideas that were true improvements to doing business!

If you have made no plans, you may have some nasty surprises waiting for you when you recover. Will it prevent your recovery? No. Can it mentally strain your recovery? Yes. Wouldn't you rather have nothing to worry about except recovering?

If you make plans, make them detailed; you may learn that the only thing your team wants from you is to butt out and let them do what you asked! If you play your cards right and plan well, you may realize that you can afford to relax more. I certainly did!

It came down to a 48-hour wait before show time.

The night before the surgery, I walked through the hardest part of all: I told my kids. If you have children, especially young ones, listen up. Talking to them about what you are facing is a very personal choice, yet the choice must be a conscious one.

I had already walked through the door of acceptance and the reward was relief. I had already walked through the door of press exposure and the reward was support and a sense of peace. Now it was time to face the toughest door yet—telling my kids I was sick. They were both under age 7 at the time.

The kids and I were just finishing our nightly ritual of brushing teeth, reading a story and saying prayers. They had no idea up to that point that anything was wrong with Daddy. After all, I still looked like a healthy bodybuilder on the outside. I still looked like Superman to them, and like most little children, they saw Daddy as the strongest man in the world who could fix anything. How to tell them that I needed to go to the hospital, but that I was going to be OK? Should I just let them have the peace of not knowing?

I reached back to my father for the answer. My father died when he was 49 years old—just 10 years older than I was at the time of my surgery. He didn't get—or listen to—his wakeup call to an unhealthy lifestyle until it was too late. He paid the ultimate price. The illness took him so fast that we hardly had a chance to say goodbye—we thought he might make it through. He waited too long to listen to his wakeup calls. We lost him so fast, it almost wasn't real. I remembered that, and I knew my kids deserved to know I was sick. In the remotely possible case that they woke up the next day without a father, I didn't want them to feel cheated because they didn't know I was sick.

I don't know how to tell anyone else to talk to their kids about a crisis they are facing, except to listen to your heart and trust your kids to understand what they need to understand.

So I decided to break it into pieces that a young child can grab and hold on to. Maybe you'll find this useful, too:

1. I told them the truth. At least in a way that was appropriate for their ages. I told them Daddy was OK, but he had a big ouchie in his belly that the doctor wanted to fix.
2. I told them what was going to happen. Daddy was going to go into the hospital for a few days, and then would come home with a big Band-Aid on his belly.
3. I gave them a sense of control. I gave them a job to do—I wanted them to write me a letter, to pray for our family and to be good for Mommy.
4. I told them what the rainbow would be after the storm. Daddy would be home with them all day for six weeks. They were so happy about that, we all almost forgot I was sick!

My oldest understood to a great extent, and was pretty quiet and reserved. My 4-year-old was a little too young to understand, which was a mixed blessing.

On the one hand, I was relieved that young age prevented my 4-year-old from worrying too much. On the flip side, I was desperately afraid that if I died, my youngest would forget me. My wife is young, and I would want her to move on and rebuild another family. But I couldn't, and still can't, spend too much time wondering if the new man of the family would become the only father my little one remembered. You think about these kinds of things, as dramatic as it may sound, when you are getting ready to go under the knife.

Why tell you all of this? I tell you because it is part of the gift of facing a crisis head on. I turned this tough hurdle into a chance to become a better father.

Only by feeling the depth of these uneasy feelings will you be able to feel the depths of love and affection that I can't even begin to describe. The love a parent has for a child defies description, and I saw the deepest reward of my crisis that night—I walked through the door of those gnawing fears, and on the other side, I found a deeper part of me, more capable of feeling and sharing the love of my family. The fear and pain are a temporary price to pay for a lifetime of deeper relationships. I can't say it any other way.

Make sure you get current with your kids, your spouse, your closest family. In the event that all doesn't go well, don't leave them saying: "If I had known he was sick, I could have said goodbye."

STEP SIX—SEE IT THROUGH

In any event in life, be it a marathon, a marriage, a divorce, the Mr. Universe competition, a track meet, or a surgery, the preparation is by far the hardest part emotionally. It is much tougher than the actual event. If you have done your homework like we have discussed so far, then the final preparations will *still* be tough. If you have *not* done your homework, the final preparations will be where you may unravel—and maybe lose the fight.

You have gone through all of the preparation and soul-searching of confronting your crisis—don't let it all fall to pieces at the starting block. Depending on your crisis, those final hours may necessitate things like intimidating medical procedures, or final confrontations with a spouse during divorce proceedings, or meeting with distraught or estranged family members to finalize a funeral. The last hours and days will contain plenty of opportunities for you to give in—to frustration, fear, anger, or hopelessness. Knowing that, part of the last step is anticipating that final stretch with— you guessed it—a plan.

The final two days before my surgery were nothing but tough final preparations.

In 48 hours, my team was going to put me under, cut me open and remove the time bomb inside me. Those were the longest two days of my life, packed with difficult medical procedures and medications, seemingly designed to knock my mental reserves down. You have to pull out all the stops to fight the drain. This is no time to turn all of your effort into a train wreck by unraveling mentally. These last hours are the quiet ones, where it is just you and your body and your mind left to do what has to be done.

This is the part that separates the survivors from the victims.

During this final stretch, you may find yourself feeling more drained than at any other time during your preparations. The physical preparation for the surgery was one of the most unpleasant experiences of my entire life. Every four hours I had to drink a fluid to evacuate my intestines, followed by a pill to control unbearable nausea. Talk about complete loss of physical control. I hadn't had that frequency of trips to the bathroom since my days at Fort Hamilton High. This time, though, I stood on a far stronger foundation.

If the final preparation to deal with your crisis includes procedures that make you feel so demoralized, degraded, or violated, be ready for it. The vast majority of people will have a huge psychological battle with themselves during that kind of preparation phase, fighting feelings of low self-worth, low self-confidence and no concept of self-love. It is *you vs. you* now.

Try to let those closest to you in, and lean on them. You must avoid the temptation to go it alone or worse—to lash out at them—when you feel miserable. This is the time to reach to your faith and to know that everything you are doing is going to make you whole again. These final hours may feel like absolute hell, but you are still a worthwhile, lovable, decent person inside. If you have to write that on a sign and put it on your wall or carry it in your wallet, do it. A steely veneer doesn't help you—or your family. In fact, it will just rob you of a golden opportunity to let God or circumstance help you strip off that veneer and let those closest to you get to know and see the real you.

I made it through that phase with a lot of leaning, a lot of self-coaching and a lot of talks with God. I had done all I could do. My action plan was set to go. My team was assembled, rested and ready. It's like when you watch a sprinter at the Olympics. He stands near the blocks in that never-ending last few minutes, when there is nothing left he can do but do it. All the preparation is done. And what will be will be.

I showed up at the hospital, nauseous, weak, dehydrated—and ready. I had the unique opportunity of having a camera crew follow me right through the doors to the admissions desk at the hospital, through pre-op and right into surgery! I'm sure I wasn't the prettiest subject the WDIV cameraman had taped in a while. He started rolling as I signed in at the nurse's station.

As exhausted as I was, I was still checking on the last minute preparations. You have to see yourself as the captain of the football team—you are in there playing hard, but you also have to make sure everyone else is ready to perform.

In the prep area, the cameraman recorded the continuing support from my family and even a final prayer with the hospital chaplain. He followed us, camera on his shoulder, and kept rolling as I was being wheeled into surgery. It was a kick to watch the tape later and see myself "checking in" with the surgical team, even as anesthesia started to kick in. One by one I looked each of the surgical team in the eye to see if they had the look of focus in their eyes. I was especially attentive to the anesthesiologist—I wanted to be sure he was "on" and ready to go. The last thing I needed was a sore back from an epidural, and I wanted him to know I wanted his best! Yeah, you could say I was trying to call the shots and lead the team right up until I lost consciousness. The camera even captured the last moment before surgery, when I grabbed my surgeon's hand and asked Dr. Bodzin and his team: "Are you ready? Did you hear me? I said, are you ready!" Team Captain to the last. Extreme? Not when you consider the extreme stakes on that table for me. It is not extreme at all for you to let your team know right up until the moment of truth that you are there to do your best, and you want their best, too.

It is *your* life in their hands—if you don't make sure that everyone is up to the task, who will? If anyone is not focused or ready, it is your job to deal with it!

BLUE SKIES AFTER THE STORM

As you might guess, I made it through my crisis—with flying colors, according to my doctors. I came out of anesthesia and I consider that moment to be the first day of a new chapter in my life.

It started out with a kiss from my wife, followed by a camera in my face. After all the effort, preparation and drama, I was the proud papa of about 12 inches of lower intestine. I got about a quick minute to rest before they wanted me on my feet.

The days are gone when a person spent two weeks flat on his back in a post-op hospital bed. These guys practically want you to walk out of surgery these days! Hey, no problem, I'm all for a quick recovery. The nurses had me out of bed and doing laps down to the nurses' station the first night. That's how you've got to take it—get right back on your feet. In my case, it was back on my feet with a nurse at each elbow. I wasn't ready to run any races yet.

My family welcomed me home, and I began my six-week recovery. Now it was time for the step that ties it all together. You have to look back and see where you've been and what it means to you. Has it changed you for the better? If you had a "negatives-to-positives" attitude, the answer is yes. So now it is time to "debrief" yourself and seize the miracle.

28

Seize the Miracle

I was alive. That is one of the sweetest feelings a person can experience—that deep gratitude just for being alive.

If you put in all that effort and make a game plan work for you, you come out better than if you'd just buried your head in the sand. Take a long moment as you enter recovery to recognize that miracle. You are officially a survivor now instead of a victim. The victims are the ones who got no warning or ignored their warnings until it was too late. You got a wakeup call in time to save your life, and you did something about it. You made it. And mental discipline, action and planning were your greatest allies. That makes you a champion. If you are like me, you also feel strongly that Someone who loves you and has a plan for you was there to guide you all along.

There will be a much-needed calm after the storm. Even the champ needs to rest! But don't lose the opportunity to ask yourself what's next. Do you just consider it a well-dodged bullet? Do you go on, business as usual, and resume the life you've been leading for 20 years up to your crisis? Can you?

If I had gotten all the way through this traumatic experience and gained nothing more than a scar, it would have been a wasted miracle. Let me explain.

As I settled into my first week at home, a deep, steady new light started to build inside me, growing stronger and brighter and warmer every day. Each time I reflected on how fortunate I was to be alive, to be healthy and happy, it grew. Each time I noticed the lack of the time-pressure burden, it grew. Each time I checked in at the club and found that all was well, it grew. Something was *different*. Even my wife noticed it.

My crisis was hard, but it was over. So *you* got knocked down? You got up again. Maybe you felt alone—but you discovered the indescribable feeling of being loved and supported by friends and family. Maybe you feel like you just got pardoned from a death sentence. I know I was knocking at death's door, and that by the grace of God, I was able to turn back. There has to be a reason for it all, a bigger lesson behind it, an opportunity you never knew you needed. That was what that growing light inside me was all about.

The name of that light is gratitude.

God had held me in my weakest hour, when I thought he might strip away everything and tear me down to nothing. I let go, made myself ready for it and was obedient to it. And when I opened my eyes, God had simply taken away the broken pieces and replaced them all with beautiful new ones. He took the injured parts of my body and allowed them to heal. He took my fears and turned them to faith. He took my worried, tense mind and gave me peace. I placed my career, my body and my life in His hands, and he reformed them and gave them back, better than before.

Will you let that happen for you? Even if you don't call it God, did you let go to something bigger than yourself—even if that's simply the collective goodwill of your support circle? Can you see what you gained by giving up what you lost? Did you gain friendships when you gave up privacy? Did you gain allies when you gave up determined independence? Did you gain a deeper love with your family when you opened your heart and leaned on them?

Getting sick again re-ignited my inner fire—my soul. It gave me the ability to see clearly three of the most important things that I have to keep at the top of my list. If this crisis is what it took for me to "get it," then it was worth every second, ten times over:

1. I am a survivor. I made it—I am not a victim, and I will never let myself be.

No matter what crisis *you* face, you have the seven steps we went through to be a survivor. Victims get hit and never get a chance to fight back. *You* are not a victim unless you choose to be, and that is a matter of action.

2. Prioritize. Ask yourself: "Are the things I am dealing with right now in my life important?" If *you* could die in the next couple of weeks, would you be worrying about the same things you are worrying about right now? Is it really important that you pass that guy in traffic that just cut you off, and end up as angry as he is? Do you really have to get to all of those business meetings at the expense of your daughter's big soccer game? Does your husband really know you love him? What will it take for you to stay focused on what is important—another crisis?

3. Let people in. I have to be *real* with myself and my family and my inner circle.

Your veneer is everyone's loss. If you chose well during your crisis, you let it strip you of your veneer and you got real and got close with the people who are important to you. Will you stay open? These days, I make sure that my family, my wife, get the *real* me. I make sure that my friends and colleagues get to see the *real* Peter, strengths and sore points alike.

All of the preparation in my life made me ready to face this crisis, and if I could go back and change it, *I wouldn't.* The Crohn's relapse was painful and frightening and disruptive to my life. It also woke me up to start taking more time for myself and my family, together. Before the relapse, you would never have caught me at home on a Saturday morning, much less a weekday afternoon. I was too busy working. Now it's a regular thing for me. Getting through my illness showed me first that I have a lot of bright, hardworking people working for me who make it unnecessary for me to be there every minute. Second, it showed me that I want *more* time with my family—every day. It brought back a lot of Technicolor into my life that had faded a bit from hard work and grueling hours. It opened me up, and I let my kids teach me how to be kid-like again. I had worked so hard for so long to be healthy enough to enjoy life. Now I've learned how to relax and *do that.* That relapse happened exactly as it was supposed to, and it turned out to be one of the most positive experiences of my life.

Crohn's disease has no known cure. My extreme attention to my nutrition and fitness goes a long way, and I am blessed with extremely long and healthy total remissions. But relapses are still a possibility. This last relapse gave me another strategy for my tool kit—I decided that on top of all the things I was already doing to take care of myself, I would take that unpleasant but lifesaving series of full gastrointestinal checks every year, instead of every five years.

Catastrophic illnesses and events are no respecters of people. One will come up and attack you and your life, no matter whether you are rich, poor, beautiful, plain, popular, shy, creative, humble, productive, black, white, female, male, straight or gay. I sincerely hope that you have your life in order and your game plan set so that you will heed the wakeup call in time to deal with it.

If you do, you are fortunate. It may sound strange, but desperation is a gift. No one knows relief like the person walking off the gallows, pardon in hand. Few experiences in this world are powerful enough to produce the profound impact that a serious crisis can have on a person. It can pluck you out of your life circumstances and give you a view from the top of the mountain, if you let it. And if you choose, you can keep the view.

Acknowledgements

This is a book, not the Academy Awards. That's good, because I need a couple of minutes to mention quite a few people who played a role in the good things that have happened to me. Life's like that if you get up off the couch and dive into each day with energy and a positive attitude. Next thing you know, you've gathered a cast of thousands.

My faith is the cornerstone of my life, something you may or may not have picked up while reading this book. My beliefs and my faith run deep. I certainly didn't try to hide them in this book, yet I respect how delicate the topic can be. Maybe someday I'll get a chance to write a book about how a muscle and fitness specialist with a successful TV and radio career—and a lingering Brooklyn accent—finds incredible strength every day in his relationship with God. For now, let me just start out by acknowledging Him.

I'd also like to acknowledge the hard work and sweat equity that the Crohn's and Colitis Foundation of America has devoted to finding a cure, providing support and allowing me the honor to serve as a national spokesperson.

Next is Jack LaLanne, who really sums up so much of what I've always wanted to be and wanted in my life: family, principle, integrity, sincerity, trustworthiness, healthy lifestyle, longevity and passion—and to be motivating and educating. I've often been heard to say that I want to be the next Jack LaLanne. Thank you for being the star that I reach for.

And, in no particular order, I need to mention a host of first-class people. Some of them you met in these pages, some of them you didn't:

Julie Levine, who showed me that it was more than a hobby.

Yvonne Wind, for wisdom beyond her years.

Robert Figliulo, one of my best friends ever and the finest mechanic on Long Island; and Walter Gatto, who was there beginning in kindergarten.

Dan Lurie, who got me to Belize.

Paul Jabara, a key link in my chain—thanks for the intro that led me to Detroit.

Tom Celani, my best friend, who—by letting me make a few bucks in endorsements—kept me alive in my early days in Detroit and who has never stopped believing in me. He is like a brother to me.

Rod Welsh, first a friend, and second, someone who made my vitamins a Blue Light Special.

Charlie Baughman, who stepped forward when things looked really grim.

Calvin Mackey, my accountant, whose numbers let me open some doors—even when I hadn't paid him yet for the numbers.

Peter Kupelian, Mark Cantor and Mark Fishman, attorneys who took care of all kinds of details that I couldn't have found with a microscope.

Chuck Robertson, for his friendship, inspiration and constant reminder that *me vs. me* is the greatest competition of all.

Cheh Low and Steven Downs of the WNBF, and Andy Bostinto of its amateur division, the NGA, for all they've done to make sure bodybuilding is about muscles and not about drugs.

Eli Zaret, Fred McLeod, Bruce Kirk and Kathy Adams—on-the-air talents who did so much off the air to make me feel at home in front of the camera.

Deborah Collura, Alan Frank, Bob Ellis and all my TV gang, for seeing and believing in my vision and passion on television.

Rich Homberg, for giving me my start in radio.

Dr. Imperato, for being the first doctor to diagnose me with Crohn's disease.

Dr. Jason Bodzin, for being used by God to help save my life with my last surgery.

Dr. Marshall Sack is one of my dearest friends. He is my doctor and my family's doctor, and I trust him with my life. I feel honored to have him as a friend.

Dr. Michael Duffy, my G.I. doctor.

John Bonner, who is my right hand and has grown into a great general manager, and to Anita Gandol, thank you for managing and training at my personal training club.

Rick Agree, who has been a great friend who I can bounce anything off of, and who I trust.

Lena Agree, my attorney.

Jackie Kallen, thank you for all your help in my early days in Detroit.

Greg Leshman and Marshall Findley, for helping me to break ground at my new Club in Southfield.

Peter Ginopolis, a great restaurateur and host—but who knows how to grill a serious whitefish without butter.

Russ Pauling, the first to license my name on a gym.